is truly the godfather of mankeps
ed all over the world

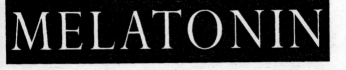

MELATONIN

▼

RUSSEL J. REITER, Ph.D.

and

JO ROBINSON

BANTAM BOOKS

New York   Toronto   London   Sydney   Auckland

MELATONIN

PUBLISHING HISTORY
Bantam hardcover edition published December 1995
Bantam mass market edition / August 1996

ISBN-13: 978-0-553-57484-5

ISBN-10: 0-553-57484-1

Published simultaneously in the United States and Canada

Bantam Books are published by Bantam Books, a division of Bantam Doubleday Dell Publishing Group, Inc. Its trademark, consisting of the words "Bantam Books" and the portrayal of a rooster, is Registered in U.S. Patent and Trademark Office and in other countries. Marca Registrada. Bantam Books, 1540 Broadway, New York, New York 10036.

PRINTED IN THE UNITED STATES OF AMERICA

OPM 10 9 8 7 6

CONTENTS

LIST OF FIGURES

FOREWORD

I first became aware of the pineal gland, melatonin, and Russel Reiter twenty-seven years ago as an undergraduate biology student. By that time, Russ and his army buddy, Roger Hoffman, had already made their first important discovery. Until they did their work, the prevailing dogma was that the pineal was a functionless, vestigial organ in the same category as the appendix. (We know better about both of these structures today!) Even though melatonin had been discovered by Aaron Lerner and his colleagues some seven years earlier, it was Reiter and Hoffman's findings that proved that the pineal actually has a significant physiological role.

In 1970, a year after my college graduation—whether through pure chance, serendipity, or as I believe, fate—I actually met Russ Reiter at the University of Rochester, while I was interviewing for a position as a Ph.D. student in the department of anatomy. When I told him that I'd done some work on the pineal in bird embryos, he invited me into his cluttered office, where he immediately started to show me his latest research data, talking with me as though I had been his scientific colleague for years, and becoming more and more animated and enthusiastic as we went on. I knew immediately that I wanted to work with him—I had been seduced! I joined Russ's group just prior to his move to the University of Texas Health Science Center at San Antonio, where I spent seven wonderful years in his lab while working on both my Ph.D. and M.D. degrees.

Although many people have been involved in unlocking the secrets of the pineal's hormone, melatonin, probably no one has been more intertwined with its research, or has made as many discoveries in this area, as Russ has. Ironically, early in his career, he was one of the most vocal skeptics about melatonin's importance. But in 1976, Russ and Larry Tamarkin, a scientist working in Connecticut, simultaneously and independently confirmed the connection between melatonin and seasonal reproductive cycles in animals. This was not only a turning point for Russ's opinion of melatonin but a major paradigm shift for the entire pineal/melatonin field. In fact, it is this very basic work that has led to current research into melatonin as a birth control agent and as a treatment for cancer—including my own findings about melatonin and breast cancer.

Russ's involvement in virtually every aspect of melatonin research, from the control of its production by the pineal gland to melatonin's actions on the various organs of the body, is indicative of his remarkable breadth of curiosity and knowledge about this fascinating molecule. Indeed, it is Russ's uncanny ability to sniff out new "hot" areas of research and to leave no stone unturned that has led him to orchestrate his most recent revolution in the field: namely, the discovery of the potent and pervasive antioxidant properties of melatonin. This discovery has new implications not only for our understanding of melatonin's role in the body but for the prevention and treatment of a variety of diseases that involve free-radical damage—including cancer, heart disease, and Alzheimer's, to name just a few.

This is where the real value of this book lies. It is about more than one man and one molecule. It is about a medical frontier that has emerged from pure intellectual curiosity about a tiny, seemingly obscure and inconsequential gland. Aided by Jo Robinson's ability to make complex science brilliantly clear, Russel Reiter tells us an exciting story about a unique substance, and about the many scientists who have dedicated themselves to finding out how it regulates the body. It is also the story of how many years of basic research are beginning to pay off, and how the results are finding their way from the researcher's bench to the patient's bedside. These discoveries are meeting the public at the very same moment as they are reaching physicians. What you will read in these pages has far-reaching implications for the body's own ability to heal itself. At the same time, it provides a responsible picture of melatonin enhancement and supplementation for those who are interested in collaborating in their own health.

For more than thirty years, Russel Reiter has been a dominant force in pineal/melatonin research. Through his unselfish mentorship, he has influenced literally hundreds of scientists working in the melatonin field all over the world today. His revolutionary vision, unbridled enthusiasm, global leadership, and dedicated work continue to pave the way for new discoveries. It is fitting that his serious yet enthusiastic voice now tells the public the melatonin story and the promises it may hold for human health.

—David E. Blask, Ph.D., M.D.
 Research Scientist
 Experimental Neuroendocrinology/Oncology
 Bassett Research Institute
 Cooperstown, New York

ACKNOWLEDGMENTS

In this book Jo Robinson and I have acknowledged some but not nearly all of the researchers who have contributed to melatonin research. Since this book is primarily related to the function of melatonin in the body, large numbers of individuals who have studied the factors that control the production of melatonin do not appear in this account. Nevertheless, we acknowledge them and their valuable contributions and thank them for what they have taught and will continue to teach other researchers.

The actual writing of the book could not have been accomplished without the support of many dedicated friends and advisers. Our agent, Richard Pine, helped shape the book and bring it to the attention of interested publishers. Toni Burbank was an extraordinary editor and supporter of the project. Crystal Eddy and Frances Robinson were with us in the trenches and are the primary reason we were able to meet an impossible deadline.

A special thank you to all the people from my laboratory who graciously gave of their time, including Burkhard Poeggeler, Dun-Xian Tan, Daniela Melchiorri, and Ewa Sewerynek. Additionally, I wish to acknowledge the intellectual support that a hundred plus postdoctoral students have given me during my scientific career. They are now pursuing science in all corners of the world. I wish I could list them all.

In addition, we would like to thank Rod Hughes for his careful scrutiny of the text; Mike Roberts, Pat McGrady, Rod Hughes, Bryan Myers, Georges Maestroni, David Blask, and Paolo Lissoni for their scientific insight; Jennifer Morris for her artwork; Bryan Burns for his graphics and on-the-spot computer expertise; Sharon Morris for her box of sharpened pencils; and Jon Sari for technical assistance. Herman Frankel and Jean Staeheli of the Portland Health Institute provided invaluable medical insight and editorial support. Finally, thanks as always to our respective spouses, Nancy Reiter and Bruce Burns, for their unflagging support.

PART I

▼

THE
LIFE-GIVING
MOLECULE

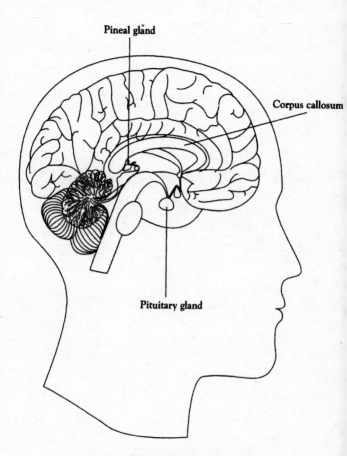

Figure 1. The Pineal Gland Lies at the
Exact Center of the Brain

CHAPTER 1

▼

MEET MELATONIN

In the exact center of your brain resides a tiny organ called the pineal (pronounced "pie-NEEL") gland, which is about the size and shape of a kernel of corn. The pineal was the first gland in your body to be formed, clearly distinguishable a mere three weeks after conception. Yet ironically, it has been the last to reveal its secrets to medical science. Thirty years ago, when I was in graduate school, I was taught that the pineal gland served no useful purpose in human beings, that it was merely a vestige of our evolutionary past. Although it had just been discovered that the gland produced a hormone called melatonin, the hormone's only claim to fame at the time was that it lightened the skin of frogs.

Today, we have begun to discover that melatonin plays multiple life-giving roles in the body. Studies conducted in my laboratory at the University of Texas Health Science Center (UTHSC) at San Antonio and in other labs around the world offer strong experimental evidence that melatonin is one of the most versatile and potent substances in the body, a principal player in the maintenance of health and well-being in all stages of life. Not only does this amazing hormone counteract stress, fight off viruses and bacteria, improve the quality of sleep, minimize the symptoms of jet lag, and regulate biological rhythms, it may even help protect against cancer, reduce the risk of heart disease, and play a role in determining how long we live.

A SUPERLATIVE SLEEP AID
AND REMEDY FOR JET LAG

Until very recently, only two of melatonin's many roles—enhancing sleep and relieving jet lag—have been highlighted in the media. The news that melatonin is an effective natural sleep aid became public knowledge in late 1993, following the announcement of results from a study conducted at the Massachusetts Institute of Technology. In this study, a group of well-rested young men were given melatonin in the middle of the afternoon and then were encouraged to take a nap. Remarkably, melatonin enhanced their sleep in a dose of only 0.1 milligrams, an amount equivalent to a few grains of salt. Articles heralding this finding appeared in newspapers around the country, including *The New York Times*, *The Boston Globe*, and *The Wall Street Journal*.

Many of the nation's 20 million insomniacs were cheered by this news, especially when they learned that melatonin is not a heavy-handed drug but a natural substance that plays a central role in the body's own sleep process. Even more appealing, a synthetic version of melatonin was available without a prescription for as little as six dollars a bottle. Despite cautionary words from some bioscientists urging consumers "not to self-medicate," tens of thousands of insomniacs gave melatonin a try. Soon it was difficult for stores to keep it in stock.

About the same time, the public learned of melatonin's ability to relieve jet lag. A number of newspapers and periodicals covered the story, including a five-page spread in the April 1994 issue of *The Condé Nast Traveler*, the bible of the jet set. Several studies had shown that melatonin dramatically reduces the symptoms of transmeridian travel. It helps people fall asleep more quickly once they reach their new destination, and even more important, it helps adjust their biological rhythms to local time. In effect, melatonin resets the body clock to match the bedside clock, cutting in half the number of days that people suffer from jet lag.

The news aroused great excitement. It wasn't long before tourists, business people, and airline flight crew were tucking melatonin into their carry-on luggage. On a recent flight to Europe I was talking about melatonin with a flight attendant. She told me about all the ways that melatonin was making her life easier. At one point she quipped, "I wouldn't leave home without it."

These two properties—enhancing sleep and relieving jet lag—quickly earned melatonin hundreds of thousands of fans. Twenty-four companies in the United States began marketing the hormone, with more coming on line every month.

Despite this burgeoning interest, however, information about most of melatonin's many talents remained hidden away in medical journals. There were two reasons for this relative obscurity. First, the discoveries were being made at such a fast pace that even we researchers had a hard time staying abreast. Second, the research was spread throughout dozens of different disciplines—cardiology, oncology, pediatrics, gerontology, chronobiology, free radical biology, immunology—and no one had bothered to assemble all the data. It wasn't until the publication of the hardcover edition of this book in 1995 that the majority of the proven and potential uses of melatonin were viewed as a coherent whole.

In the chapters that follow, I will explore melatonin's

many properties in detail. But first, I want to give you a brief overview of some of the most notable findings.

FAST-BREAKING DISCOVERIES

▶   MELATONIN BOOSTS THE IMMUNE SYSTEM

In recent years, immunologists have vastly expanded our understanding of the immune system. They've discovered how immune cells "talk" to each other, how they inhibit and stimulate each other to insure a comprehensive defense, among many other things.

But without melatonin, the picture is incomplete. One of melatonin's main functions, we have recently learned, is to trigger the body's nightly cycle of rest and repair. As you will see in more detail, melatonin is produced primarily at night. At around two or three in the morning, when your melatonin levels peak, there is a significant increase in the number of immune cells circulating in your bloodstream, enhancing your body's defenses against cancer, viruses, and bacteria. New research shows that melatonin may play a direct role in this heightened activity.

Melatonin also plays a vital role in boosting your immune system when you are under stress, whether that stress comes from viral infection, emotional stress, drugs that suppress the immune system, or the aging process.

Immunologists are now investigating dozens of potential uses for melatonin. In the near future, people may be taking it to speed the healing of wounds, enhance the effectiveness of vaccines, fight off colds and fevers, counteract the toxicity of chemotherapy, offset the immunosuppression that accompanies surgery, and jump-start an aging immune system.

▶ MELATONIN IS THE MOST POTENT, VERSATILE ANTIOXIDANT

As a nation, Americans toss down almost a billion dollars' worth of the antioxidant vitamins each year. We eat foods high in antioxidants and take antioxidant vitamins because studies have shown that they give us a wide range of health benefits, from a lowered risk of heart disease and certain cancers to a reduced incidence of cataracts. Antioxidants help protect us from disease by attacking dangerously reactive molecules called free radicals, which can cause extensive damage to the body. More than sixty diseases, from rheumatoid arthritis to herpes zoster, are now believed to be caused or exacerbated by free radicals. Antioxidants stop free radicals in their tracks, helping to preserve the integrity of our cells and protect our overall health.

What you may not realize is that your body produces its own antioxidants, which play an even more vital role in protecting you from free-radical damage. In 1993 my colleagues and I at UTHSC discovered that melatonin is the most potent and versatile of all the known antioxidants. This discovery has profound implications for human health and longevity.

▶ MELATONIN PROTECTS AGAINST ENVIRONMENTAL HAZARDS

We live in a toxic world. The air we breathe, the water we drink, and the food we eat are all contaminated by herbicides, pesticides, toxic waste products, and a vast array of other potentially lethal substances. Many of these toxins wreak their havoc by generating free radicals. At UTHSC we have shown that melatonin provides an unprecedented level of protection against these environmental hazards. New evidence suggests that melatonin can also protect the body from self-inflicted toxins such as alcohol and tobacco.

▶ **MELATONIN HELPS MAINTAIN A HEALTHY HEART**

In recent years medical science has made great strides in reducing the death rate from heart disease. Most of these gains have been made by perfecting surgical interventions and by designing drugs that reduce high blood pressure and cholesterol. Still, despite these advances, heart disease remains the number-one killer of both men and women throughout the industrialized world.

Recent research has given us new insight into one of the body's own mechanisms for maintaining a healthy heart—the nightly production of melatonin. Melatonin lowers cholesterol and blood pressure, researchers have found, and reduces the risk of irregular heartbeat. In one pilot study, melatonin normalized the blood pressure of people with hypertension within a week, with no negative side effects.

▶ **MELATONIN MAY HELP PREVENT CANCER**

Compelling new evidence suggests that melatonin plays a primary role in the body's defense against cancer. In a number of studies, when animals were protected with melatonin before being injected with a potent carcinogen, cancer failed to develop.

Melatonin may also slow the growth of cancer once it is established. Test-tube studies have demonstrated that melatonin inhibits the growth of a number of human cancer cells, including breast cancer, lung cancer, cervical cancer, melanoma, and most recently, prostate cancer. These findings are beginning to be tested in human studies. So far, melatonin has prolonged the survival and improved the quality of life of hundreds of people with terminal cancer.

▶ **MELATONIN AUGMENTS OTHER CANCER THERAPIES**

Melatonin shows even more promise in treating cancer when it is used in combination with other therapies. In pilot studies conducted primarily in Europe, melatonin has improved the effectiveness of virtually all forms of cancer therapy, including chemotherapy, surgery, immunotherapy, and radiation. When melatonin is added to these therapies, more patients experience complete remission of their tumors than when these therapies are used alone. In addition, the majority of patients live longer, experience fewer side effects, and have a better quality of life. The clinical implications are enormous.

▶ **MELATONIN MAY BE A POWERFUL WEAPON AGAINST AIDS**

Hundreds of millions of dollars have been spent on AIDS research, but efforts to find a cure or develop an effective vaccine have been frustrated at every turn. So far, the successes have been limited to delaying the progression of the disease and improving the treatment of the many opportunistic diseases that can accompany the illness.

Melatonin may prove to be a worthy adversary of the AIDS virus. It stimulates a number of immune cells known to be deficient in AIDS patients (including T-helper cells, natural killer cells, and a vital signaling compound called interleukin-2). In addition, melatonin has the potential to protect AIDS patients from the toxic effects of frequently prescribed drugs such as AZT and to improve the quality of life of those in the final stages of the disease.

►   **MELATONIN HAS LITTLE OR NO TOXICITY**

What sets melatonin apart from virtually all other treatments for cancer and AIDS is its lack of toxicity. Hundreds of animal and human studies have shown it to be an extremely safe, nontoxic, and nonaddictive hormone. In the most extensive trial to date, fourteen hundred women have been taking high doses of the hormone for over four years with little evidence of negative side effects. Dozens of smaller studies have produced similar findings. According to one knowledgeable researcher, "You'd have to drown yourself in melatonin to have it be toxic."

►   **MELATONIN PROMISES TO ADD YEARS TO YOUR LIFE AND LIFE TO YOUR YEARS**

Taking melatonin may extend your healthy, productive life span. As you age, your body produces less and less melatonin, depriving you of this sleep-enhancing, free-radical-scavenging, heart-calming, immune-stimulating, cancer-fighting hormone—in short, depriving you of one of your best defenses *against* aging. Replenishing your supply of this vital hormone may allow you to live longer and delay the onset of crippling diseases such as arthritis, diabetes, heart disease, cancer, Alzheimer's, and Parkinson's. This possibility is more than wishful thinking. In laboratory studies, giving melatonin to aging animals has extended their life span by as much as 20 percent.

MELATONIN—INEXPENSIVE AND AVAILABLE

The fact that a substance with so many remarkable properties is available for sale without a prescription is unprecedented in the annals of medicine. Nor to my knowledge, has a substance of this import ever been marketed at such an early stage of the research. Most of the studies to date have involved small numbers of people. In fact, some of the research is still at a basic level, which means test-tube and animal experiments but not yet human studies. We have a great deal yet to learn about melatonin, including which doses are best for which uses and who should *not* be taking it.

The potential downside of melatonin's new-found popularity was brought to my attention just a few days ago while I was listening to a health segment on a local radio talk show. A caller was asking for help in getting her five-year-old daughter to take a nap. I was amazed to hear the doctor advise her to give the little girl melatonin. "It's a natural sleep aid," said the doctor, "and it has no toxicity." That much is true. But what the doctor must not have realized is that the body produces very little melatonin in the daytime. If you take a melatonin tablet at the wrong time of day, you work at cross-purposes to your natural biological rhythms. Even more troubling, children produce ample amounts of melatonin on their own. Except in rare instances—and then only under a doctor's supervision—there is no reason to give children melatonin.

Despite this downside, I disagree with some colleagues who urge that melatonin be pulled from the stores. From all we know, melatonin appears to be a safer product than many of the medications currently being sold, from aspirin to FDA-approved prescription drugs. *But if melatonin is to remain available to the public, it must be used responsibly. And if people are to use it responsibly, they need accurate information about its properties, as well as reliable advice about how to use it appropriately.*

Until now, it has been difficult for the lay public to get the detailed information they seek. A number of patients have discovered that they know more about melatonin than their physicians. Others have been given erroneous information by their doctors. For example, one woman told me that her psychiatrist advised her not to bother to take melatonin as a sleep aid. "It's a protein," he told her, "and like most proteins, it won't be absorbed into the bloodstream intact. It will do no good." The doctor gave her a prescription for a potent sleep medication, instead.

In truth, melatonin is *not* a protein, and it enters the bloodstream with ease. Something else the psychiatrist didn't know is that the medication he prescribed *blocks* the body's production of melatonin, interfering with the body's natural sleep mechanisms. Because of the widespread use of melatonin and the lack of knowledge of its properties, accurate, authoritative, and up-to-date information about melatonin is urgently needed.

ABOUT THIS BOOK

As I talk to more and more people about melatonin, I sense a major shift in popular thinking about health care. Many people no longer believe that their family physician has the answers to all their health questions. In their passion to get well or stay well, they are pursuing medical information on their own, through magazines, books, excursions on the Internet and by braving the scientific literature itself.

This book offers a brand-new area of medical knowledge for you to explore, one that has the potential to enhance your health and longevity in ways never before possible. Melatonin can do much more than give you a good night's sleep or ease the transition from New York to Rome—it may rewrite the program of planned obsolescence that is built into your genes. As you read about the research that backs up this provocative statement, you will be faced with a monumental question: Should you join the hundreds of thousands of others taking part in this anti-aging experiment, or should you acquiesce to the natural aging process? For the first time in history, you may now have a choice.

This book is divided into three parts. In Part I, I will take you on a medical mystery tour, explaining what we know about melatonin and how we learned it. This forty-year saga required researchers to solve some unusually difficult problems. The insights that have resulted from this ambitious campaign, I believe, are among the most significant to come from any field of medical research.

Along the way, you will learn a great deal about how your body keeps you healthy and whole. Absorbing some of this information will challenge you to master new terminology and to expand your knowledge of human physiology. I chose not to simplify the subject matter any more than I have, however, because I believe the information will prove invaluable to you, helping you to become a more informed consumer of health products and, even more important, a more knowledgeable participant in your own health care. It is my hope that you will share in some of my own excitement about melatonin and gain, as I have, a renewed reverence for the human body.

Part II contains information about protecting your body's production of melatonin. Your natural supply of melatonin is vital to your health because it helps your body function the way it was *designed* to function. A modern lifestyle may be robbing you of this important hormone. For example, in our ignorance—and arrogance— we have constructed artificial lighting environments that alienate us from the earth's natural cycle of light and dark. This artificial lighting can wreak havoc on your production of melatonin, giving you too much melatonin in the daytime, when you want to be active and alert, and too little at night, when you need to be sleeping.

Electromagnetic fields (EMFs)—those invisible waves of energy given off by power lines, household wiring, and electrical appliances—may also be reducing your melatonin levels, a possibility that is now being scrutinized in laboratories around the world. But the worst threat to your natural supply of melatonin may be to take one of many common prescription drugs. Drugs that have been proven to lower melatonin levels in humans include the most widely sold pain relievers, a popular anti-anxiety drug, the top-selling antidepressant, and many heart medications. Chances are great that you or someone you love has recently taken a substance that interferes with their production of melatonin.

Also in Part II, I will explain natural ways to stimulate and supplement your production of melatonin. Making only a few changes in your eating habits and daily routine may cause a significant rise in your nighttime melatonin levels. Even if you decide not to take melatonin supplements, you may still be able to give yourself the melatonin advantage.

Part II will also answer questions commonly asked about taking melatonin supplements. It lists possible negative side effects and explains why some people should refrain from taking melatonin altogether. I will discuss the different kinds of preparations now available and highlight the benefits and drawbacks of each. Throughout the book I will be discussing currently recommended doses and protocols for treating a variety of conditions, including insomnia, jet lag, shift work, cancer, and AIDS, so you can share this information with your doctor. If you want to do further reading—and I encourage you to do so—all the main points in this book are referenced in notes at the end.

Part III will give you a glimpse into the future of melatonin research. I will present preliminary data suggesting that melatonin may help prevent or alleviate diabetes, the fourth leading cause of death in the United States. I will also explain exciting new work by child specialists showing that the hormone may have beneficial effects on children suffering from autism or epilepsy or who are at high risk for sudden infant death syndrome (SIDS).

This paperback edition concludes with a special supplement in which I answer the most commonly asked questions about melatonin. Following the supplement is a brief survey for melatonin users. By participating in this survey, you will be making a valuable contribution to our understanding of this amazing molecule.

CHAPTER 2

▼

THE THREE-BILLION-YEAR-OLD MOLECULE

"How can one molecule have so much influence on health and well-being?" is a question I am frequently asked. We researchers have been asking ourselves the same question. Now we have a theory that explains the hormone's multiple actions. The theory hinges on the fact that melatonin is a very old molecule. It has been found in every animal and plant studied to date, from human beings to the most primitive one-celled algae that evolved more than three billion years ago. In each organism, melatonin's molecular structure is identical; the melatonin circulating in your veins is chemically the same as that extracted from algae, plants, insects, frogs, and seals.

This sameness is a rare occurrence in biology. Only a limited number of substances are common to all life-forms in precisely the same molecular configuration. Without exception, all these substances have been found to be essential to life as we know it.

Something else unusual about melatonin is that in all

the life-forms in which it has been studied, the hormone has been produced in the same circadian (more or less day-long) rhythm, with higher levels produced at night than during the daytime. This production cycle is common to animals, plants,[1] and even algae.[2] It is possible that all living creatures share this daily ebb and flow of melatonin, an internal tide that protects and heals.

The fact that melatonin is a universal substance, that its molecular structure is unchanging, and that it has the same circadian rhythm throughout the plant and animal kingdoms led researchers to conclude that melatonin plays a fundamental role in the biology of all cells. But before I tell you what that role is, I'm going to give you a few highlights of the forty-year odyssey that led researchers to this conclusion, in the order in which the findings were made.

A FOUR-YEAR SEARCH FOR THE SKIN-LIGHTENING FACTOR

Many scientific breakthroughs require insight, hard work, and blind luck. Aaron Lerner, M.D., a Yale dermatologist, needed an extra helping of all three in order to discover melatonin. The year was 1953 (I was yet in high school), and Lerner was searching for the hormone that lightens human skin. He was interested in a skin condition called vitiligo, which is characterized by patches of depigmented skin. He had already discovered the hormone that darkens skin, which he named melanocyte-stimulating hormone, or MSH. Now he was hot on the trail of the skin-lightening hormone. An abnormal production of this hormone, he thought, might be responsible for vitiligo.

Lerner searched the scientific literature for information about potential skin-lightening compounds and turned up a vital clue: According to an obscure 1917 article, the pineal gland might produce a hormone that blanches the skin. In the article, two scientists reported that they had dumped ground-up cattle pineal glands into a tank filled with tadpoles. They were surprised to see that in thirty minutes, the skin of the tadpoles had become transparent, making visible their hearts and intestines. As far as I know, the scientists never tried to find out whether the pineal extract did anything for the cows from which it came, or if the tadpoles produced any of the stuff on their own. And for the most part, nobody cared. The small size of the pineal gland and the lack of evidence that it played a meaningful role in animals, much less humans, made it a dead-end area of research.

But now, Lerner had reason to be interested in the gland: Did *human* pineal glands produce a skin-lightening factor as well? If so, would inhibiting its production help treat vitiligo? To answer these questions, he first had to isolate the exact substance that had blanched the tadpole skin. Unbeknownst to him, this skin-lightening agent would prove to be elusive indeed.

Lerner and several colleagues proceeded to amass thousands of cattle pineal glands and submitted them to an elaborate, time-consuming purification process. The bean-sized glands were freeze-dried, cleaned of extraneous tissue by hand, pulverized, defatted, then rehydrated in a Waring blender. This low-cal extract was then centrifuged, concentrated, filtered, mixed with solvents, evaporated, and combined with ethanol. It took 2,500 pineal glands to produce a hundred milligrams of the dried extract—about the amount of salt you'd sprinkle on an ear of corn.

But their work was only just beginning. Their next step was to isolate the precise *molecule* responsible for the lightening effect. They separated the extract into various fractions using a technique called chromatography. Then they applied each fraction to a piece of stretched frog skin to see if it lightened the skin. The active part of the pineal extract, they discovered, was an extremely small portion of the whole. If the compound turned out to be a hormone, which they assumed it would, it was produced in smaller amounts than any known hormone.

The researchers had no choice but to repeat the complicated process over and over again. This is "bench work," the tedious, unglamorous labor that occupies much of a researcher's time. As Lerner sat hunched over his bench—cleaning, filtering, weighing, centrifuging, evaporating—he had at least one comforting thought. He was stalking his quarry in peace—this was no Crick-and-Watson race to the finish line. As far as he knew, he and his colleagues were the only scientists in the entire world interested in pineal extracts. "It was not a competitive field," he remarks dryly.

It took almost four years, but eventually the Yale researchers managed to work their way through a quarter-million cattle pineal glands—a Herculean task. Unfortunately, the compound was present in such infinitesimal quantities that all of those glands netted them a mere 0.00000353 of an ounce, little more than "an invisible layer of molecules on the bottom of an otherwise empty flask."[3] In order to produce the 10 milligrams that they needed for determining its molecular structure, they would have to purify the pineal glands of more than a million cattle. Daunted, they decided to abandon the extraction project.

Still, Lerner found that he couldn't turn his back on all that effort. He would give himself an additional four weeks, he decided, to gather up all the clues they'd uncovered to see if he could figure out the extract's molecular structure through logic. If he could come up with a hypothetical molecular structure, he would be able to mix up a test compound and compare it with the actual pineal extract. If the two substances had identical properties, he would know he had guessed correctly.

After two weeks, Lerner had an insight that allowed him to guess at the chemical formula of the skin-lightening hormone.[4] He called his colleague Jim Case, and the two of them hurried to the lab to mix up a batch of the test compound. With growing excitement, they compared it with the pineal extract. They were one and the same. The riddle was solved.

Lerner had discovered a brand-new and extremely potent hormone, the most potent one he had ever tested. (He found it was a hundred thousand times more effective at lightening frog skin than adrenaline.) He gave the hormone the official designation N-acetyl-5-methoxytryptamine, but he also blessed it with a more melodious name: melatonin. He chose *mela* because the hormone lightens the cells that produce the pigment *mela*-nin, and *tonin* because the hormone is derived from the chemical sero*tonin*.[5]

Lerner published his findings in 1958 in a one-page article in *The Journal of the American Chemical Society*. Eight years later, when I was beginning my own career as a melatonin researcher, I looked up Lerner's article. I was struck immediately by the brevity of the report. Lerner gave no indication of the prodigious effort that had gone into isolating and identifying melatonin, and there was no hint of its future significance. For such an important hormone, it was an inauspicious beginning.

TOXICITY TESTING

Once melatonin had been properly categorized and christened, Lerner and other scientists began exploring what else it might do, other than blanch frog skin. But first they had to see if it had any toxic effects. In 1960, Lerner injected melatonin into the first human subject. He administered what would be a megadose by today's standards—200 milligrams—but he observed no negative side effects other than a "mild sedation."[6] Later, he injected melatonin into a number of patients with skin diseases to see if it would help them. Alas, human skin did not respond. All of Lerner's efforts had been for naught. Reluctantly, he abandoned melatonin and went on to more promising areas of research.

A number of other researchers became interested in melatonin, however, if only because it was new and unexplored territory. It's not every day, after all, that a new hormone is discovered. At the National Heart Institute in Bethesda, Maryland, scientists had enough curiosity about melatonin to subject it to a standard toxicity test. In this test, increasing amounts of a substance are injected into rodents until half of them die. This final dose is known as the LD_{50}, which stands for "the lethal dose for half of the population." (Regrettably, scientists do not know how to determine the toxicity of a substance in a test-tube experiment; they must observe its effects on living creatures.) Try as they might, the researchers could not determine the LD_{50} for melatonin, even though they injected mice with as much as 800 milligrams of it per kilogram of body weight, which for adult humans would be equivalent to injecting a half-cup of pure melatonin. Even this massive dose "failed to produce death" in the animals.[7] The scientists attempted to give the mice even higher amounts, but they could not force any more of the hormone into solution.

SEARCHING FOR THE "HIBERNATION FACTOR"

I entered the scene in 1964, having just graduated from the Bowman Gray School of Medicine with a Ph.D. in endocrinology. I was spending two years fulfilling my military requirement in the U.S. Army Medical Service Corps, where my supervisor was a civilian researcher, Roger Hoffman, Ph.D. Hoffman was assigned to a project that sounds like something straight out of *Star Trek*—he was trying to find a way to put future astronauts into suspended animation. The military had ambitious plans to send astronauts to distant planets (perhaps because the Soviets had gotten ahead in the space race by launching Sputnik), and it was looking for some way to save food and energy on the long voyages. If army researchers could figure out what triggered hibernation in animals, the process might be adapted for future space travelers.

Hoffman and I never did solve all the riddles of hibernation, but we did make a discovery that stimulated considerable interest in the pineal gland. Through our work with hibernating hamsters, we learned that melatonin triggers the seasonal breeding of animals. It was the first conclusive evidence that the pineal gland plays a meaningful role in *any* species, a discovery that coincides with the beginning of the modern era of melatonin research.

A TRANQUILIZING, SLEEP-INDUCING HORMONE

But what does melatonin do in humans? We're not seasonal breeders (or so it seemed at the time), yet we too produce melatonin. One of the reasons researchers were so slow to identify melatonin's roles in the body is that the amounts present in the bloodstream are so small that until the 1970s we could not measure them. It was difficult to measure *any* hormone with accuracy, because they are such potent substances that they are eked out in nanograms—billionths of a gram. Melatonin, however, presented an even greater challenge because it is produced in picograms—*trillionths* of a gram!—the smallest amount of any known hormone. Thus we had no idea how much melatonin humans produced or when they produced it—a major roadblock to understanding the hormone.

Lacking this technical ability, researchers tried to gain insight into melatonin's actions by injecting humans with a synthetic version of it. (The body may produce very small amounts of melatonin, but using Lerner's formula, an ambitious chemist can mix up copious quantities in a few days.) Volunteers were injected with varying doses and watched closely for reactions. Throughout the early human studies, the hormone was found to have tranquilizing, sleep-inducing properties. This reaction was clearly evident in a study conducted in 1970 by a Mexican researcher named Ferdinando Anton-Tay, M.D. Anton-Tay recruited eleven volunteers and hooked them up with various devices so he could measure their brain waves, respiration, and heart function. Then he injected them with as much as 75 milligrams of melatonin. Within minutes of receiving the injections, the patients began producing slower brain waves—a sign of tranquillity. Soon most of them were sound asleep. When Anton-Tay awakened them about forty-five minutes later, they reported having unusually vivid dreams and experiencing a sense of "well-being and moderate elation."[8]

This study and similar ones showed that melatonin has many of the opposite effects of adrenaline. Adrenaline increases the heart rate, tenses the muscles, raises the blood pressure, and compels one to take action. By contrast, melatonin lowers the heart rate, relaxes the muscles, and lulls one to sleep. If adrenaline is the "fight-or-flight" hormone, then melatonin is the "rest-and-recuperate" hormone.

THE CHEMICAL EXPRESSION OF DARKNESS

Melatonin research moved a giant step forward in the mid-1970s, with the development of a new technique for measuring biological substances when they are present in very small quantities. The technique is called radioimmunoassay, or RIA. The development of RIA is to endocrinologists, it has been said, what the development of the telescope was to astronomers. Thanks to RIA and other even more accurate processes, researchers were able to measure accurately the amount of melatonin present in the human bloodstream. Within the space of a few years, information was collected about melatonin levels in hundreds of volunteers.

Out of this data came a crucial finding: Humans produce five to ten times more melatonin at night than during the day, a circadian rhythm found in animals as well.

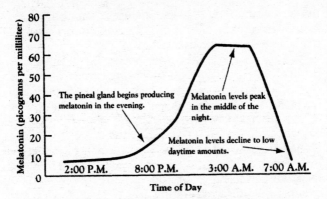

Figure 2. The 24-Hour Cycle of Melatonin Production

Daytime levels of melatonin are very low. Nighttime levels may be 5 to 10 times higher. (Note that these amounts are given in picograms, *trillionths* of a gram, per milliliter of blood.)

We produce our peak amounts around two or three in the morning. This strong nighttime surge has earned melatonin the nickname "the chemical expression of darkness." This insight helped us home in on melatonin's role in the body. Researchers began to ask, How does human physiology differ from day to night? Is it possible that melatonin helps bring about some of those changes?

MELATONIN THROUGHOUT THE LIFE CYCLE

As researchers pondered these questions, we learned another key fact about melatonin: Production of it varies considerably over the life span. Newborns produce very little melatonin, we found, until around three months of age. Three months happens to be the stage of development when they begin to sleep longer stretches at night and to be more alert during the daytime. We began to suspect that melatonin might be the underlying reason for this regularity. Once babies produce a strong nocturnal surge of melatonin, they have a hormonal pacemaker that helps them tell night from day.

Babies produce increasing amounts of melatonin, we learned, until they are about one year old. Then their nocturnal melatonin levels remain steady until just before puberty, when they decline markedly, a trend that continues for the next five years or so.[9] This steep decline got us to wondering if a falling concentration of melatonin helps trigger the onset of puberty.[10] In animals, high levels of melatonin are known to inhibit reproduction. Do human melatonin levels have to go down before we become sexually mature? Some researchers argued they do, while others shot the notion down.

The most recent studies suggest a strong tie between melatonin levels and sexual maturity. For example, children who are late to enter puberty have been found to have higher levels of melatonin than their peers.[11] Correspondingly, children who enter puberty extremely early (as early as three years of age) may produce only a third as much melatonin as other children their age.[12] Having the right amount of melatonin at the right stage of life appears to be one of the keys to normal sexual development.

A number of years ago, I was called in as a consultant in the case of a young man in his mid-twenties who had yet to go through puberty. His sexual organs and overall appearance were characteristic of a fourteen-year-old boy, not a man well into adulthood. Two endocrinologist friends, Dr. Manuel Puig and Dr. Susan Webb, had given the patient the usual hormonal treatments, but none of them had had the desired effect. Further investigation revealed that the young man had melatonin levels five times higher than normal. Over the next few years, his melatonin production began to wane. Whether this happened spontaneously or in response to the hormones he was given is not known. But when his melatonin levels dropped to the level of a normal preadolescent, he finally entered puberty. Eventually, he married and was able to father a child.[13]

MELATONIN CONTINUES
TO DECLINE WITH AGE

For those of us who have successfully navigated adolescence, it is of far greater significance that melatonin may also trigger *senescence*. As you can see in the graph in Figure 3, the body's production of melatonin declines inexorably with age. A seventy- or eighty-year-old may have the hormone in amounts so small as to be undetectable.

A number of hormones decline with age, including testosterone, estrogen, growth hormone, and DHEA (dehydroepiandrosterone), which is a precursor of the sex hormones. The gradual loss of these hormones was once seen as a *consequence* of aging, but now researchers are beginning to suspect their loss may *contribute* to the aging process, and that replacing them may extend our youth. Preliminary studies suggest that they are right. But of all the hormones, melatonin appears to have the greatest

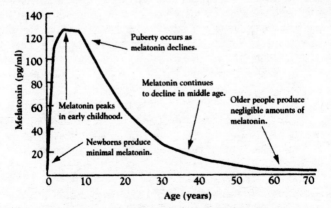

Figure 3. **Nocturnal Melatonin Levels Throughout the Life Span**

This graph shows peak nighttime levels of melatonin throughout the human life span. Melatonin levels are relatively high in early childhood and decline from adolescence onward.

anti-aging potential, a subject to be explored in Chapter 12.

MELATONIN STIMULATES THE IMMUNE SYSTEM

One of the reasons that melatonin has so many rejuvenating powers is that it protects and enhances the immune system, especially in aging organisms. This property came to light in the 1980s, largely through the efforts of my friend and colleague Georges Maestroni, Ph.D., director of the Center for Experimental Pathology in Locarno, Switzerland. Maestroni became interested in melatonin's role in the immune system in 1977. In a systematic, step-by-step campaign, he and his colleague Ario Conti, Ph.D., expanded the way we view the immune system.

Maestroni, Conti, and another colleague, Walter Pierpaoli, demonstrated many of their theories by conducting rodent experiments. Early on, they demonstrated that when mice were deprived of their normal supply of melatonin, they were less able to fight off disease. But to Maestroni, this finding was ambiguous. Perhaps the methods they had used to block melatonin production—raising the animals in constant light or injecting them with melatonin-lowering drugs—had been stressful to the animals, and stress all by itself can cripple the immune system.

So, in 1984, Maestroni moved on to what he hoped would be a more definitive test of melatonin's effect on the immune system: he would inject the hormone into healthy rodents to see if it *increased* their immune response. He and his colleagues divided twenty mice into two groups. One group was injected with melatonin and the other with an inactive saline solution. A day later, all the mice were injected with cells from sheep—cells that their immune systems would recognize as intruders and fight off. After six days, the researchers counted the number of activated immune cells in each of the mice. Maestroni discovered that the melatonin-treated mice had substantially more activated immune cells. He called out to Conti, "This is it! We were right!" They found that the mice treated with melatonin had 133 percent as many activated immune cells as those that had not.

It was the defining moment of Maestroni's long exploration. In the following years, his studies would produce results much more dramatic than this one. For example, he and Conti would show that melatonin keeps mice from dying from a deadly virus, that it counteracts the toxic effects of chemotherapy, and that it may reduce the severity of type I diabetes in mice. Yet of all his studies, he told me, this one humble experiment had the greatest emotional impact. After seven years of theorizing and preliminary studies, he finally had definitive data showing that melatonin enhances the immune response of at least one species of animal.

For a medical researcher, nothing compares with the moment of discovery. For a short amount of time, you are the only human being alive to know this one new fact about the world. You have extended human knowledge, if only by one small observation about the immune system of mice. Maestroni, however, had an immediate sense of the greater implications of his finding. If he could show that this inexpensive, nontoxic hormone stimulates the immune system of *humans as well*, then the practice of medicine might change just as dramatically as it did in the 1940s, when sulfa drugs and penicillin were introduced.

DISCOVERING MELATONIN'S ANTIOXIDANT PROWESS

Eight years later, in 1992, I had one of my own moments of discovery. Ever since 1958, when Lerner discovered melatonin, it had been fixed in everybody's mind that melatonin was a hormone. We had no idea back then that melatonin was leading a double life—now a hormone, now an antioxidant. No one had explored this possibility because no other hormone was known to have this dual capacity; antioxidants were antioxidants and hormones were hormones, and never the twain shall meet. But melatonin turned out to be an exception to the rule.

As happens in many scientific discoveries, we stumbled upon melatonin's antioxidant role while we were trying to answer an entirely different question. Melatonin influences an enzyme inside heart cells, we knew, but we couldn't figure out how, since these heart cells have no melatonin receptors. We knew that hormones don't cause changes inside a cell unless those cells have the right kind of receptor. It's an inviolable rule of hormones—no receptors, no reaction. Yet melatonin was clearly altering the level of this enzyme.[14]

We were stymied. Then we turned up a clue. This particular enzyme, we learned, could be influenced by the amount of free radicals in a cell. If the amount of free radicals changed, the level of the enzyme changed. We knew that one way to change the amount of free radicals is to expose the cell to an antioxidant. Was it possible, we wondered, that melatonin influenced the enzyme by interacting with free radicals? In other words, was melatonin *an antioxidant as well as a hormone*?

We decided to find out. Two of my post-doctoral fellows, Dun-Xian Tan and Burkhard Poeggeler, exposed a dilute solution of hydrogen peroxide (the same stuff you have in your medicine cabinet) to ultraviolet light generated by a high-tech sun lamp. This simple procedure generates a wealth of free radicals. Through a complicated (and expensive) process, they figured out how many free radicals it created. Then they repeated the experiment with melatonin added to the solution. They discovered that melatonin got rid of a large percentage of the free radicals. It was *indeed* an antioxidant.

After three more years of research, I can now say with confidence that melatonin is not just an antioxidant—it appears to be the most efficient and versatile antioxidant known. It is twice as effective as vitamin E, five times as

efficient as glutathione, and five hundred times more effective than the synthetic antioxidant DMSO.

A THREE-BILLION-YEAR LEGACY

At the beginning of this chapter, I proposed that melatonin must perform a function that is vital to the survival
of all living organisms. Paradoxically, melatonin's most
recently discovered role—protecting organisms from free-
radical damage—appears to be its original and most fundamental role, one that it may have been performing for
several billion years.

To understand this concept, you need to have a sense of
how life on earth evolved. Aeons ago when the earth was
formed, there was no free oxygen on the planet. The beau-
tiful, blue-skied, watery world that we know today was a
steamy, sulfurous, volcanic, barren planet. Then after a
few millennia, one-celled creatures appeared that did not
need oxygen to survive. Instead, they used energy derived
from the sun in a primitive version of photosynthesis to
draw carbon and nitrogen atoms directly from the atmosphere. These atoms became the raw materials they
needed to sustain life. After a time, more sophisticated
cells evolved that were able to use water as part of their
photosynthesis process. A waste product of this more refined photosynthesis process was oxygen. Gradually these
primeval life-forms multiplied, and oxygen accumulated in
the atmosphere. The process of photosynthesis converted
an atmosphere with virtually no free oxygen to one that is
now 21 percent oxygen.

To oxygen-breathing humans, this sounds like a step in
the right direction. But the original anaerobic (without
oxygen) creatures could not survive in an oxygen environment. They were replaced by the aerobic (with oxygen)
organisms. Still, even to aerobic organisms, oxygen turned
out to be a good-news-bad-news substance. The good news
was that oxygen allowed them to make more efficient use

of organic molecules like glucose. The bad news was that in the process, free radicals were formed that had the capacity to deform molecules, perforate cell membranes, and damage DNA. In order to survive, organisms had to develop some form of protection against them, and the best protection was to manufacture an antioxidant. Melatonin appears to have been one of the first molecules to excel at the job.[15]

As time passed and aerobic organisms became more complex, melatonin continued to perform this vital function. It had no choice, because antioxidants are bound by the laws of physics to react with free radicals. Melatonin gets rid of or scavenges free radicals whether it meets up with them in a biologist's test tube, the leaf of a plant, or the eye of a human. Once an antioxidant, always an antioxidant.

Over time, however, melatonin inherited additional roles. After all, it had a couple of billion years in which to take on the occasional odd job. In more complex lifeforms, melatonin began to function as a hormone as well. Thus, in the human body, melatonin is both a superlative antioxidant and a master hormone. This unique combination of functions is the primary reason that melatonin has so much influence on your health and well-being.

CHAPTER 3

▼

THE BEST ANTIOXIDANT

"Too many free radicals, that's your problem."
"Free radicals, Sir?"
"Yes. They're toxins that destroy the body and brain—
caused by eating too much red meat and white bread
and too many dry Martinis."
"Then I shall cut out the bread, Sir."

James Bond in *Never Say Never Again* (Ian Fleming, 1983)

Right now, as you read this page, melatonin in your blood is preventing the oxidation of LDL cholesterol, the "bad" cholesterol that can clog your arteries. Melatonin in your brain is safeguarding your irreplaceable neurons from free-radical attack. Melatonin in the fluid within your eyes is helping to prevent free radicals from forming cataracts. Melatonin in the lining of your gut is reducing your risk of ulcers. Every cell in your body is vulnerable to the attack of free radicals, and every cell in your body is protected by melatonin. Without protection from melatonin and a host of other antioxidants, you would die within a matter of hours.

Our understanding of the role that free radicals play in our health is just as recent as our understanding of melatonin, and for much the same reason—until this decade, scientific technology was inadequate to the task. As mere fragments of molecules, free radicals are so small that we cannot see them, not even with an electron microscope. Furthermore, they are such extremely reactive substances that they come into being and then disappear in the space of a nanosecond, a billionth of a second.

Within this decade, free-radical biologists have devised ingenious ways to monitor free-radical damage as it occurs, giving us a *molecular* view of disease and aging. Their research suggests that free radicals cause or exacerbate a rogue's gallery of diseases including cancer, AIDS, asthma, adult respiratory distress syndrome, cataracts, emphysema, fetal alcohol syndrome, heart disease, macular degeneration, stroke, ulcers, Alzheimer's, Parkinson's, and rheumatoid arthritis. Furthermore, researchers have produced convincing evidence that free radicals play a major role in the aging process itself.[1]

DESPERATELY SEEKING AN ELECTRON

So what are free radicals? How do they wreak their havoc? As you probably recall from high school biology, a molecule is composed of two or more atoms held together by electrons, which revolve in separate orbits. Ideally, each orbit contains an even number of electrons, which balances out the molecule's electrical charge and stabilizes the entire structure. A free radical is different from other molecules in that it has an unpaired electron in its outer-

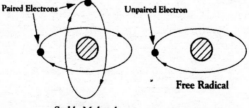

Figure 4. **What's Different About Free Radicals?**

most orbit. This may sound like a trivial distinction, but a molecule with an unpaired electron is unstable and is compelled by the laws of physics to steal an electron from another molecule, or else to burden another molecule with its spare electron. This is not just a molecular game of hot potato. Electrons are the flexible atomic glue that holds a molecule together. So when a free radical interferes with the electrons of another molecule, it will deform, corrode, or otherwise destroy it. On the cellular level, this interference destroys cell membranes, disables vital enzymes, and corrupts the genetic code. To an organism, this could mean disease or even death.

WHERE DO FREE RADICALS COME FROM?

Many of the free radicals that assault your cells are an inevitable consequence of breathing oxygen. Oxygen is vital for your survival because it converts carbon-rich molecules into the energy you need to sustain life. However, the part of the cell that produces this energy, the mitochondria, does not operate flawlessly. As much as 5 percent of the oxygen taken into the mitochondria "leaks out" in the form of oxygen-based free radicals, which amounts to a staggering one trillion free radicals per cell per day.

Another source of free radicals is the immune cells. Various immune cells generate the noxious molecules to use as weapons against viruses, bacteria, and cancer cells. Ideally, they deliver the free radicals in a surgical strike, causing little damage to surrounding tissue. But during an all-out bacterial or viral invasion, your immune cells produce vast amounts of free radicals, which can injure healthy cells. AIDS, rheumatoid arthritis, and toxic shock are believed to be exacerbated by this inadvertent free-radical damage.

Free radicals are also formed in abundance by exposure to external hazards such as ultraviolet (UV) light, sulfur dioxide, ozone, tobacco, alcohol, wood smoke, asbestos, pesticides, herbicides, solvents, and radiation. The proliferation of these hazards may help explain the dramatic increase in cancer rates in the industrialized world. In Russia, which has a long legacy of environmental neglect, the life expectancy of men has fallen to 57.3 years, fourteen years fewer than men in the United States. According to a 1995 article in *The New York Times*, "scientists are looking more closely at the history of Soviet ecological abuse for answers."[2]

THE EVERYDAY DAMAGE
CAUSED BY FREE RADICALS

You could live in a cabin in the Swiss Alps and dine on organic vegetables, however, and still die from free-radical damage. The main difference is that you would die a slower and less painful death. Simply breathing oxygen and being exposed to the radiation of the sun burdens your body with free radicals. Over time, the damage adds up. We call this damage aging.

You may not notice the external signs until you reach middle age. Then you might wake up as I did one morning and suddenly notice age spots dotting your hands and face—a sign that free radicals generated by UV light from the sun cause the development of a skin pigment called lipofuscin. Or you might see a candid photograph of yourself and be shocked to discover that your jowls are beginning to hang in soft crepey folds—visible evidence that free radicals have been undermining the collagen proteins that support your skin.

As disconcerting as these blatant signs of aging may be, the erosion that has been taking place *within* your body is of far greater consequence. All the time that free radicals have been making inroads into your vanity, they have been busily laying the groundwork for cancer, eroding your brain cells, sabotaging your liver, clouding your vision, and destroying microscopic amounts of heart muscle. In effect, they've been shortening your remaining days on earth one molecule at a time.

TO THE RESCUE—MELATONIN AND OTHER ANTIOXIDANTS

Fortunately, you are not defenseless against this onslaught. Your body is rich in antioxidants, substances that have the ability to stop free radicals from forming or to limit the damage they cause. Antioxidants get their name because they combat oxidation. (Oxidation is a reaction in which a molecule loses an electron. Thus, when a free radical pirates an electron from an intact molecule, it is said to *oxidize* that molecule.)[3]

There are two major sources of antioxidants: those that you get from food or food supplements (vitamins E, C, and beta-carotene, for example), and those that are produced within your own body. The antioxidants you produce inside your body are less well known but just as vital. They include molecules such as glutathione and uric acid, which scavenge free radicals directly, and antioxidative enzymes such as glutathione peroxidase, catalase and superoxide dismutase (SOD), which break them down into nontoxic products. Melatonin is a new star on this scene.

HOW MELATONIN MAY PREVENT CANCER

We are now in the process of discovering the extent of melatonin's remarkable antioxidant properties.[4] Of all the antioxidant experiments we've conducted at UTHSC, the one that had the most impact on me was the very first one, in which we demonstrated that melatonin could protect living creatures from cancer.

Free radicals play a major role in the initiation of many cancers. The process in many cases begins when free radicals cause significant damage to the DNA molecule, the large double-stranded molecule in the nucleus of a cell that contains the instructions for the creation and functioning of the entire organism, including that particular cell. DNA is a very large molecule, which means that it has a lot of surface area vulnerable to attack by free radicals. It has been estimated that by the time you are seventy years old, the DNA in each of your cells has sustained hundreds of thousands of direct hits from free radicals.

The vast majority of these hits cause minor damage that is repaired before the cell has a chance to divide. But the odds are great that the DNA molecule in at least one of your trillions of cells will sustain extensive free-radical damage that goes unrepaired, resulting in a mutant cell. It takes but one of these cells to seed a malignant tumor. No wonder autopsy reports show that half of all people seventy and over have a tumor lurking somewhere in their bodies!

At UTHSC, my postdoctoral fellows and I found that melatonin may help prevent cancer by serving as DNA's personal bodyguard. We made this discovery by injecting rats with safrole, a toxic substance known to cause cancer by unleashing large amounts of free radicals. We injected half of these rats with melatonin as well. Twenty-four hours later, we examined their liver cells for DNA damage. The animals that had been given safrole alone had sustained significant damage to their DNA; if the experiment had continued, many of them would have developed liver cancer. Careful measurements revealed that the DNA of the melatonin-treated rats had sustained only 1 percent as much damage. (See Figure 5.)

I was astounded by these results. Most scientific studies produce barely significant results. Scientists long for those rare studies that provide dramatic evidence—what we call

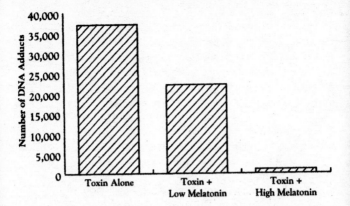

Figure 5. Melatonin Protects DNA from Free-Radical Damage

Melatonin protected DNA from the toxic effects of the cancer-causing agent safrole. The more melatonin, the greater the level of protection. The high dose of melatonin prevented 99% of the damage.

a robust effect. Well, this was a robust effect if we had ever seen one. In fact, my initial thought was that something must have gone wrong with the experiment, and I suggested that we do it again. We got the same results the next time, and the next. As the significance of the study began to sink in, I was awestruck by the apparent potency of melatonin. We had given the animals *750 times* more of the toxin than melatonin, yet the hormone had offered near total protection.[5]

MELATONIN PROTECTS AGAINST RADIATION

Another experiment that was of special interest to me is one in which we showed that melatonin protects human white blood cells from radiation. Preventing radiation damage is a stiff challenge for any antioxidant. Radiation creates free radicals by ripping apart benign water molecules (H_2O) and converting them into hydroxyl radicals ($OH^•$). The hydroxyl radicals, the most destructive of all the free radicals, proceed to rob electrons from nearby molecules, setting in motion a devastating chain reaction. Molecules that have been deprived of their electrons yank electrons from their neighbors, and on and on until the body is consumed in a molecular wildfire. It was a torrent of hydroxyl radicals that killed the Soviet workers exposed to the blast of radiation from the Chernobyl nuclear power plant disaster of 1986.

To see if melatonin could prevent this type of free-radical damage, my colleagues and I exposed human white blood cells to radiation. At the conclusion of the experiment, we found that melatonin protected the cells better than any other known antioxidant. Remarkably, it was *five hundred times* more effective than the synthetic antioxidant DMSO, which is regarded as an excellent radioprotector.[6]

This finding has obvious practical applications. The last time you were given an X-ray or mammogram, you probably noticed that the X-ray technician stepped out of harm's way before activating the machine. That's because no amount of radiation has been found to be absolutely safe. In the future, you may be asked to take a melatonin tablet before being given a diagnostic X-ray, giving you the equivalent of an internal lead apron.

MELATONIN PREVENTS CATARACTS IN ANIMALS

In 1993 a postdoctoral student named Mitshube Abe, M.D., was working in my lab. Abe's field was ophthalmology, and he wanted to see if melatonin could protect the eyes from free radicals. The lens of the eye is approximately 98 percent protein. When the protein becomes damaged by free radicals, it coagulates, making it opaque. The result is cataracts. (This is very similar to what happens when you fry the white of an egg.) The older you are, the longer your eyes have been exposed to UV light from the sun, and the more likely you are to have cataracts.

Somehow your body "knows" that your eyes are vulnerable to free-radical damage, and it provides them with an extra helping of antioxidants—a built-in pair of sunglasses. Melatonin is especially abundant in the eye. As you age, however, you produce less and less melatonin, which may make you more and more vulnerable to cataracts.

Abe worked with a group of young rats that had been depleted of their supply of glutathione, one of the important antioxidants produced in the body. (Like melatonin, glutathione has been found in virtually all organisms.) Young rats that are made glutathione-deficient form cataracts in as little as two weeks. We gave half of these rats melatonin to see if it could prevent them from forming. Sixteen days later, we examined the animals and found that the rats that were not given melatonin had cataracts in both eyes; in the melatonin-treated group, only one rat had a cataract, and that was just in one eye.

This is another study with obvious clinical applications, as Abe suggests in a recent paper:

> Considering that senile cataracts in the human are
> considered to be the result of oxidative stress . . .
> it is possible that supplementing elderly individuals
> with melatonin, which is normally lost during aging, may delay and/or prevent cataract development normally associated with aging.[7]

A number of studies are now under way to see if other antioxidants can reduce the risk of cataracts. Melatonin deserves this scrutiny as well. In the meantime, people who have been taking melatonin for other reasons have found that their eye health has improved. For example, I heard from a woman from Portland, Oregon, who had cataracts in one eye. Her vision was so impaired that she was unable to drive safely at night. She began taking melatonin as a sleep aid and found that her eyesight improved. She can now drive at night with little difficulty.

FREE RADICALS AND THE BRAIN

Of all the organs in the body, the brain is the most vulnerable to free-radical attack. Your brain, which constitutes only 2 percent of your body weight, consumes 20 percent of the oxygen you inhale, subjecting it to a steady stream of free radicals. Your brain is especially susceptible to damage because of its high concentration of unsaturated fatty acids—complex molecules that are easy targets for free radicals because they have a "loose" hold on their electrons. Also, brain tissue is rich in iron, which can transform hydrogen peroxide, a by-product of oxygen metabolism, into hydroxyl radicals.

Free-radical damage is devastating to the brain because the neurons, the nerve cells in the brain, do not regenerate. The brain cells that are helping you read this text are the very same cells you were born with, except that they've sustained a great deal of damage in the interim. Once you lose a certain percentage of neurons, every aspect of your mental functioning is compromised, from memory to motor control. Free-radical damage is now believed to play a formative role in most brain disorders, including Alzheimer's disease, Lou Gehrig's disease, multiple sclerosis, and Parkinson's disease.[8] The chances are great that if you live long enough, you will have one or more of these diseases. Surveys show that half of all centenarians are afflicted with Alzheimer's disease.

A possible way to prevent these neurodegenerative diseases is to take antioxidants. But the brain presents a unique challenge. So essential is the brain to survival that it is shielded by a special barrier called the blood-brain barrier. This barrier screens out some (but unfortunately not all) harmful substances and helps maintain a very delicate balance of chemicals and other substances. Regrettably, this barrier also denies the brain access to most antioxidants. Researchers have spent millions of dollars trying to design synthetic antioxidants that can enter the brain in sufficient quantities to prevent neurodegenerative diseases.

Evidence shows that melatonin crosses the blood-brain barrier with ease. We demonstrated this fact in our most recent antioxidant experiment, in which we found that melatonin protects the brain from free radicals generated by stroke. Strokes occur when blocked arteries prevent the flow of oxygen-rich blood to the brain. Brain cells that are deprived of oxygen for a period of time will die, causing significant damage to the brain. But additional damage occurs when the artery is unblocked and blood *returns* to the brain. This process unleashes a great many free radicals, producing a secondary damage called reperfusion injury. Reperfusion injury can be even more damaging to the brain than the initial stroke.

In our experiment, we successfully protected rats from reperfusion injury by treating them with melatonin. This result suggests that people who have just suffered a stroke might fare much better if they, too, were treated with the antioxidant-hormone.

MELATONIN IS THE MOST POTENT AND VERSATILE ANTIOXIDANT KNOWN

In addition to the experiments I've mentioned, my group at UTHSC has shown that melatonin prevents free-radical damage caused by the toxic pesticide paraquat; protects the stomach from the corrosive effects of alcohol; and prevents damage caused by the bacterial toxin (LPS) that causes toxic shock and sepsis. Whenever we have pitted melatonin against a free-radical foe, melatonin has been the winner by a knockout.

In the process, we have gained a great deal of insight into melatonin's antioxidant properties. Here is what we have learned:

▶ MELATONIN IS A GLOBAL ANTIOXIDANT

Free radicals damage surrounding molecules in a nanosecond. Unless an antioxidant is in the immediate vicinity, they cannot be prevented from doing so. Thus, an antioxidant must offer "on-site" protection. But most antioxidants cannot do this. For example, vitamin C is water soluble, which limits it to fluid environments such as the cytosol, the watery interior of the cell. Cell membranes are fatty molecules; taking vitamin C to protect them would be like trying to put out a fire in the attic when the fire extinguisher is locked in the garage. Melatonin is both fat and water soluble—a rare occurrence in nature—making it the only known antioxidant that can protect all parts of the cell.[9] Furthermore, because melatonin can navigate all the barriers in the body with ease, including the blood-brain barrier and the placental barrier (which protects the unborn child), the antioxidant-hormone can protect every cell in the body.

▶ MELATONIN IS A VERY POTENT ANTIOXIDANT

Compared on a one-on-one basis, melatonin may be at least twice as effective at protecting cell membranes as vitamin E, formerly regarded as the body's premier fat-soluble antioxidant.[10] It is five times more potent than glutathione in neutralizing hydroxyl radicals.[11] Remarkably, it is *five hundred times* more efficient at protecting cells from radiation than DMSO, which is known for its radioprotective qualities.[12]

▶ **MELATONIN DOES NOT PRODUCE
    FREE RADICALS**

A number of well-known antioxidants can actually *create* free radicals under certain circumstances. Vitamin C, for example, has a Jekyll-and-Hyde personality. Most of the time it is an excellent antioxidant, but when it is exposed to free iron—which can happen whenever your tissues are damaged by heat, trauma, infection, radiation, or toxins—it can assist in the creation of free radicals. Melatonin has never been shown to generate free radicals.

▶ **MELATONIN HAS NO KNOWN TOXICITY**

Some antioxidants can be toxic in excessive amounts. The synthetic antioxidants BHA and BHT, widely used as food preservatives, have known cancer-promoting abilities in animals and may interfere with your body's blood-clotting ability.[13] Excessive amounts of selenium, an essential component of the antioxidant glutathione peroxidase, can cause your hair and fingernails to fall off. Other antioxidants interfere with the cells' ability to generate energy. Beta-carotene in excess can cause nausea or vomiting.

Even some of the antioxidants you produce within your body can be harmful under certain circumstances. For example, people with Down syndrome have an extra copy of the gene that produces the antioxidant enzyme SOD, resulting in unusually high levels of the substance. This overabundance of SOD creates large amounts of hydrogen peroxide, which, in the presence of iron, can be transformed into hydroxyl radicals. Damage from hydroxyl radicals may account for the premature aging and shortened life span of people with this common genetic disorder.

Melatonin appears to have none of these drawbacks. It has little or no toxicity, not even in megadoses; it does not interfere with energy generation; and it does not produce hydrogen peroxide or hydroxyl radicals under any known circumstances.

▶ **MELATONIN OFFERS SPECIAL PROTECTION
    TO DNA**

We have recently learned that melatonin is found in especially high concentrations in the nucleus of cells.[14] Inside the nucleus, it forms a close association with the DNA molecule. Just exactly how melatonin links with DNA is not yet known, but test-tube and animal studies have shown that melatonin has an unparalleled ability to protect DNA molecules from free-radical damage. Even in the very small amounts produced within the body, the hormone offers substantial protection.[15] Its ability to safeguard DNA may make melatonin a key factor in cancer prevention.

▶ **MELATONIN CAN BE ADMINISTERED ORALLY**

Melatonin is easily synthesized and can be administered in a great variety of ways including by tablet, injection, nasal spray, skin cream, and transdermal patch. Most other endogenous antioxidants are not effective when administered by these methods. Furthermore, once in the body, melatonin does not have to be converted into some other form, so you don't have to worry about having the right enzymes or "co-factors." Thus, if you wish, you can easily augment your natural supply of melatonin with a convenient, inexpensive supplement.

CHAPTER 4

▼

BOOSTING THE IMMUNE SYSTEM

In recent years, the news has been full of accounts of new and deadly diseases—AIDS, Ebola virus, Marburg virus, Hanta virus, drug-resistant pneumonia, drug-resistant tuberculosis, flesh-eating bacteria. These diseases strike a note of horror in us for two very good reasons: They can be lethal, and they are difficult or impossible to cure. The only good to come out of these diseases is that they have focused attention on the immune system as never before. Hundreds of millions of dollars have been funneled into immunological research, greatly increasing our knowledge of the body's healing system. This research may soon pay dividends, not only in combating these deadly diseases but in helping us defeat garden-variety cold and flu viruses as well. It may even help us triumph over the one infirmity we share in common—the gradual crippling of the immune system that comes with age.

A highly significant but unheralded finding to come out of this flurry of research is that melatonin is a dominant player in the immune system. The discovery is only a few years old, but researchers are already demonstrating melatonin's ability to treat cancer, slow the progression of AIDS, make the body more resistant to colds, and protect the immune system from the toxic effects of chemotherapy.

THE MULTILAYERED IMMUNE SYSTEM

The recognition of melatonin's role in the immune system is part of an overall expansion in our concept of immunity. Back in the 1960s, the immune system was thought to embrace a large assortment of immune cells plus a few key organs such as the spleen, thymus, bone marrow, and lymph nodes. Little was known of how intimately the immune system interacts with other systems such as the endocrine (hormonal) system and the nervous system.

Today the immune system is viewed as a global enterprise, incorporating every aspect of the body. Of particular interest is the relationship between mind and body, or in medical terms the nervous system and the immune system. Studies have shown that you can influence your health by practicing meditation or visual imagery, having a deep religious faith, belonging to a supportive network of family and friends, or learning to think more positively.[1] Even fleeting emotions can boost your immunity, a fact that can be verified under a microscope. In a recent study, groups of volunteers were shown either of two documentaries: one an uplifting film about Mother Teresa, and the other a comparatively bland nature film. Blood samples were drawn from the volunteers before and after each viewing. The volunteers who watched the inspiring story about Mother Teresa had a significantly greater increase in white blood cells than those who watched the nature film.

Correspondingly, negative thoughts and feelings have been shown to have a *negative* impact on your health. Statistically, people who have been recently widowed are more likely to die in the year following the death of the spouse. More recently, people infected with HIV who show signs of depression have been found to have a poorer prognosis than those who do not.[2] The fact that depressed people are more vulnerable to disease may be due, in part, to the fact they have a deficiency of "natural killer cells," a class of immune cell that protects the body against cancer and viruses.[3]

How do moods, those ephemeral blends of thoughts and feelings, influence immune cells? Our understanding is incomplete, but researchers have discovered that certain immune cells have receptors (or docking stations) for neurotransmitters, the substances that transmit impulses between nerve cells and play a determining role in one's state of mind. (Serotonin and dopamine are examples of neurotransmitters.) When you are depressed, a deficiency of neurotransmitters interferes with the flow of messages between your brain cells. As a result, you feel sluggish and unmotivated and have less ability to experience joy. This same deficiency of neurotransmitters is detected by your immune cells, and in ways not fully understood, it results in a *depressed* immune system as well as a depressed mood.

HORMONES AND YOUR HEALTH

Hormones also have a significant impact on health. Testosterone, which is considered a male sex hormone because it is more abundant in men than in women, actually *inhibits* the immune system. In a number of studies, male animals that have been castrated (which eliminates the production of testosterone) had a lower incidence of disease than did intact animals. They also lived longer.[4] The same may be true for human males. In a bizarre experiment conducted in the 1950s in a mental institution in Kansas, a number of male patients were castrated to see if it made them more tractable. (Testosterone is associated with aggression, and scientists hoped that lowering the

testosterone levels of the men would eliminate some undesirable behavior.) Whether the men were any easier to
manage is not known, but they did live longer and healthier lives. In fact, they outlived the clever researchers who
devised the experiment, the uncastrated male patients,
and most of the female patients.

Estrogen, a hormone that is more abundant in women
than in men, plays a complex role in the immune system.
It reduces a woman's risk of acquiring some diseases but
increases her risk of acquiring others. Women as a group
are more resistant than men to infectious diseases, but
they are more likely to be afflicted with autoimmune diseases. Women have twice the rate of multiple sclerosis,
three times the rate of rheumatoid arthritis, and nine
times the rate of systemic lupus, a disease that attacks the
connective tissues of the body. Immunologists believe
these diseases are related to estrogen because they wax and
wane along with fluctuations in blood levels of the hormone.

Stress hormones are without gender bias—they occur
in both men and women and dampen the immune response of both. You may have noticed that when you are
under prolonged stress, you are more likely to get sick and
may take longer to recover. Both physical and mental
stress increase your production of a hormone called cortisol. Your immune cells have receptors for cortisol, and
when cortisol links with those cells, it slows down their
rate of division, leaving your immune system short-
handed.[5]

Intuitively, it would seem that a weakened immune system might make it more difficult to survive a stressful
episode. But the net effect of the stress hormones is to
enhance your survival. When you are under acute stress,
the stress hormones divert your energy away from nones-
sential functions such as reproduction and the healing
process and toward your muscles; when you are running
away from a predator, you don't want your body to be
preoccupied with fighting off a minor cold or distracted by

thoughts of mating. When the crisis is over, you will have plenty of time to attend to these everyday matters.

ENTER MELATONIN

That melatonin plays a central role in the body's immune system is a fact that eluded most melatonin researchers, myself included, until the mid-1980s. Between 1965 and 1985, I must have conducted hundreds of experiments in which animals were either injected with melatonin or deprived of the hormone by having their pineal glands removed (a procedure called pinealectomy). My interest at the time was in reproduction, not immunology. But I saw no clear-cut evidence that either an abundance or absence of melatonin had a significant impact on their health.

In hindsight, I now know why we were so slow to catch on to melatonin's immune-enhancing effects: They are most evident when animals are under stress. I'm using *stress* here in the broadest sense, to include physical stress, psychological stress, environmental stress, and the stress that comes from disease and aging. For the most part, the animals we were studying were living remarkably stress-free lives. We obtained the rats when they were young and in prime condition, so they showed none of the chronic stress that comes with aging. We fed them a high-quality rat chow that helped maintain a strong immune system. (You and I would be far healthier if we dined on an equivalent "human chow.") The temperature and humidity in the animal room were carefully controlled, protecting the rodents from environmental stress. Finally, because of strict legislation governing the treatment of laboratory animals, the room was kept cleaner than a suite at a four-star hotel. We were forbidden even to place charts on the walls, lest they provide hiding places for cockroaches.

All told, the rats experienced far less stress than they would have in the wild. They had no need to hide from enemies; no reason to forage for food; no exposure to inclement weather, and less contact with dust, bacteria, vermin, and viruses than those of us who were studying them. The only significant stress in their lives was confinement and boredom.[6]

MELATONIN BUFFERS THE EFFECTS OF STRESS

Under more normal conditions, we now know, the amount of melatonin in an animal's bloodstream can mean the difference between life and death. The researcher who opened our eyes to this reality is Georges Maestroni. One of the findings that piqued his interest back in 1977 was that when animals' pineal glands were removed, their thymus glands shriveled up. It had been known since the early 1960s that the thymus is essential for a vigorous immune response. Maestroni reasoned that if a healthy thymus gland requires the presence of melatonin, then melatonin must also be vital to the immune system.

Step by logical step, Maestroni has proven this theory correct. A study he published in 1988 showed the dramatic effect that melatonin can have on the immune system.[7] In this study, Maestroni, Ario Conti, and Walter Pierpaoli injected a group of mice with a sublethal dose of a virus called the encephalomyocarditis virus, or EMCV. As a rule, healthy young rodents will fight off the disease, but mice that have weakened immune systems due to stress or aging will die from it.

After injecting the mice with the virus, Maestroni and co-workers stressed them by confining them for several hours a day in individual tubes perforated with air holes, a procedure called restraint stress. Being confined in the tubes did not harm the mice physically, but it did make them anxious, and anxiety generates stress hormones, which cause a significant decline in the immune response.

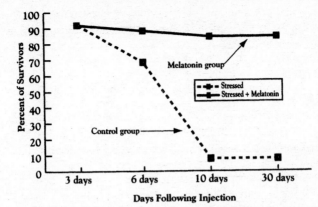

Figure 6. Melatonin Protects the Immune System from Stress

Two groups of mice were stressed and then injected with a virus.
One of the groups was protected with melatonin. A much higher
percentage of the melatonin-treated rodents survived.

Then the researchers injected a portion of the mice with
melatonin to see if it enhanced their survival.

The mice were observed for the next thirty days. A
high percentage of the ones that had not been treated
with melatonin died within the first week of the experiment. Meanwhile, most of the melatonin-treated mice
managed to fight off the virus *even though they had been
subjected to the same amount of stress!* At the end of the
study, 82 percent of the melatonin-treated mice had survived, compared with only 6 percent of those not given
the hormone—a striking difference in mortality.

MELATONIN BOOSTS
THE IMMUNE SYSTEM OF HUMANS

Clearly, a life-and-death study such as this will never be
conducted on humans, but unwittingly you and I may be
guinea pigs in a similar experiment. It takes little imagination to see the parallel between Maestroni's mice-in-the-

tube experiment and riding in a subway car or airplane crammed with kids with runny noses and adults who are sneezing and hacking—the mix of confinement, stress, and exposure to viruses is the same. Will taking melatonin supplements help us ward off disease?

According to preliminary studies, the answer is yes. In a double-blind study conducted by Virginia Utermohlen from Cornell University, ten male college students were given either 20 milligrams of melatonin or a placebo each night for one week. The next week, they received the alternate treatment. It just so happened that a virus was going around the campus at the time of the study, and most of the men who participated had colds. While they were taking melatonin, they produced 250 percent more salivary IgA, a protein in the saliva that helps protect against colds and upper respiratory infections.[8]

WHAT IS A DOUBLE-BLIND STUDY?

A double-blind study is one in which a treatment such as melatonin is compared with a placebo (a substance or treatment known to have little effect) or to an alternative treatment. *Double-blind* refers to the fact that neither the researchers nor the subjects know which treatment they are receiving. This type of study has been shown to produce more objective and repeatable results than ones in which the researchers or subjects are aware.

In 1995, Italian researchers showed that melatonin can also boost the immune system when people are under extreme stress. The study subjects were twenty-three cancer patients who were undergoing traditional cancer therapy. As many people can attest, the diagnosis of cancer in and of itself can produce a great deal of stress. When this psychological stress is coupled with the negative side effects of radiation, chemotherapy, and/or surgery, the result can be a severely depressed immune system.

To see if melatonin could protect the immune systems of these patients, the researchers gave them 10-milligram tablets of melatonin each night for a period of a month. They found that melatonin increased production of parts of the immune system known to be essential in the body's fight against cancer. (Specifically, the patients had a 28 percent increase in tumor necrosis factor alpha, a 41 percent increase in interferon-gamma, and a 51 percent increase in interleukin-2.[9])

MELATONIN PROTECTS THE IMMUNE SYSTEM IN OLD AGE

Stress and aging have a number of similar effects on the body. In both instances, the body produces more stress hormones, the thymus gland shrinks or involutes, and the number of immune cells declines. In particular, older people as a group have a deficiency of vital immune cells called T cells, and the T cells that they *do* produce are less capable of doing their job. (The T cells of older people produce half as much interleukin-2, or IL-2, as those of younger people. IL-2 is essential for stimulating other immune cells.[10] Thus, a deficiency of T cells can impoverish the entire immune system.)

Health statistics attest to the fact that the immune system declines with age. A teenager has 1 chance in 25,000 of dying of cancer, and only 1 chance in 2 million of dying from an infectious disease other than AIDS.[11] By contrast, a person seventy or older has a 1-in-8 chance of dying of cancer and a 1-in-30 chance of dying of an infectious disease.[12]

Can melatonin help reverse this age-related decline in immunity? The animal research gives us reason to hope. In 1992 three researchers from the University of Rome gave melatonin to a group of one-year-old mice. (Mice are such short-lived creatures that their immune system begins to decline at six months of age.) The mice were injected with red blood cells from horses. Their immune system would bombard these foreign cells with disease-fighting proteins called antibodies. Half of the mice were then injected with melatonin. After four days, the researchers counted the number of antibodies in both groups of mice. The melatonin-treated mice were producing more than twice as many antibodies as the untreated mice—proof of a more aggressive immune response.[13]

A more recent study suggests that melatonin may be even more effective in protecting the immune system of older animals than younger animals. In this 1995 experiment, both young and old mice were injected with a virus that causes encephalitis, an often fatal brain infection. Half of each group was then treated with melatonin. In the mice not given melatonin, 6 percent of the young ones and none of the old ones survived the deadly disease. In the melatonin-treated group, 39 percent of the young mice and a surprising 56 percent of the old mice survived.[14] These findings offer new hope that old age and infirmity need not go hand in hand.

HOW MELATONIN INFLUENCES SPECIFIC PARTS OF THE IMMUNE SYSTEM

Today, research into melatonin's role in the immune system is progressing very rapidly, with new insights being published every month. These findings have allowed us to see how melatonin influences individual components of the immune system, bringing us one step closer to developing therapies to prevent or treat specific diseases.

From an immunologist's point of view, perhaps the most significant finding to date is Maestroni's and Conti's 1995 discovery that melatonin causes many of its actions by linking with a type of cell known as the T-helper cell.[15] To immunologists, this discovery is like being handed a road map after being lost for days in a strange country. Now they can apply all that they know about T-helper cells to their observations about melatonin.

T cells are among the most important cells in the immune system. They originate in the bone marrow and then migrate to the thymus gland (thus the T), where they are trained to respond to a particular target. One T cell may be subtly altered so that it responds to the polio virus, another to hepatitis-B, a third to the AIDS virus, and so on. Each T cell has a unique target. When a T cell graduates from the thymus, it goes on the prowl for its enemy. Right now you have billions of T cells in your body on the lookout for their individual targets. Once a T cell spots its enemy, a complex process is set in motion that results in the production of millions of clones. Thus your body can go from having a single scout to a well-equipped army in a matter of days.

You produce two main types of T cells: T-killer cells, which are a part of the attack team, and T-helper cells, which direct the whole operation. T-helper cells coordinate other cells in the immune system by producing a family of intercellular signaling substances called cyto-

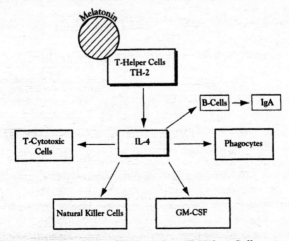

Figure 7. Melatonin Stimulates T-Helper Cells

kines. Each cytokine regulates a different set of cells, suppressing the growth of some and stimulating the growth of others. (Cytokines include the interleukins, interferons, colony-stimulating factors, and tumor necrosis factors.) Without T-helper cells coordinating the immune system, the battle would be lost. It would be as if you were trying to fight a war when your entire communication network has broken down.

Maestroni's and Conti's breakthrough discovery is that there are melatonin receptors on T-helper cells. When a cell has a receptor for a given hormone, it implies that the hormone plays a significant role in regulating that cell. The Swiss researchers have shown that when melatonin docks with its receptor on the T-helper cell, a cascade of events is set in motion, starting with the stimulation of a factor similar to a key cytokine known as interleukin-4, or IL-4. This IL-4-like factor, in turn, stimulates a group of other immune components. As you can see, when melatonin links with a T-helper cell, ripples are sent out to a great many parts of the immune system. In the following pages I will discuss how your health is influenced by just three of those components—natural killer cells, phagocytes, and GM-CSF.

▶ MELATONIN STIMULATES NATURAL KILLER CELLS

As you can see by Figure 7, one type of cell that is stimulated by melatonin is the natural killer cell, or NK cell. NK cells specialize in attacking two of your body's stealthiest invaders—cancer cells and virus-infected cells. These particular enemies are very difficult for your surveillance system to detect because they camouflage themselves as healthy cells. Viruses hide deep within a cell, commandeering its internal machinery to make clones of themselves, leaving few traces on the outside of the cell to betray their presence. Cancer cells are just as devious in that they retain virtually all the external markings of the healthy cells from which they sprang. Identifying a virus-infected cell or a malignant cell is like trying to distinguish between friend and foe on a battlefield when both sides are wearing the same uniform. Fortunately, your NK cells have mastered the art.

Taking small amounts of melatonin can cause a dramatic increase in your production of NK cells. In a study published in 1994, six healthy young men took 2 milligrams of melatonin each night for a period of two months. Their NK cells were measured before and after the study. At the end of the treatment period, the men were producing an average of 240 percent more NK cells, more than doubling their arsenal against cancers and viruses.[16]

▶ MELATONIN STIMULATES PHAGOCYTES

Another phenomenon triggered by melatonin is the enhancement of the killing power of a voracious family of

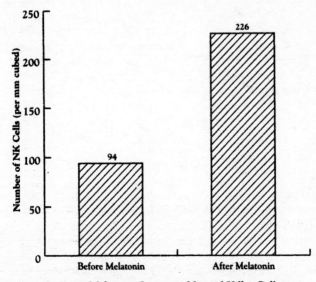

Figure 8. Melatonin Increases Natural Killer Cells

cells known as phagocytes. The word *phagocyte* (pronounced "FAG-o-site") means "eater (*phago*) of cells (*cytes*)," an apt description for these hungry creatures whose primary job is to ingest and digest the enemy. Typically, phagocytes are the first to arrive on the scene of a viral or bacterial invasion and the last to leave. When they identify their targets, they send out long protuberances that entrap the invaders and draw them into their shapeless bodies. They engulf the attackers, isolate them in fluid-filled pockets called vacuoles, then assault them with syncopated bursts of free radicals and noxious chemicals.

When all the enemies are destroyed, the phagocytes move on to their next job—cleaning up the debris. So zealous are phagocytes in their efforts that, if the situation warrants, they will ingest so many of the enemy that they burst. Pus, the yellowish fluid that accumulates at the site of an infection, is strewn with the carcasses of kamikaze phagocytes.

A study published in 1994 revealed that melatonin enhances the killing power of a particular phagocyte called a monocyte. Researchers at Northwestern University Medical School in Chicago withdrew monocytes from human volunteers and incubated them in a dilute concentration of melatonin—in fact, the approximate concentration that can be found in your bloodstream late at night. This trace amount of melatonin increased the ability of the monocytes to destroy skin cancer cells by 73 percent.[17]

▶ MELATONIN STIMULATES GM-CSF

All of the trillions of white and red blood cells in your body originate from the same mother cells, called uncommitted stem cells, which make their home in your bone marrow. If all of your immune cells were destroyed with the exception of your stem cells, it would be theoretically possible to replenish all the cells.

Maestroni and Conti announced in 1995 that melatonin promotes the growth of bone marrow cells.[18] There are many instances when the ability to stimulate bone marrow cells would prove invaluable. One obvious instance is during chemotherapy. Most of the drugs used to destroy cancer cells are toxic to the bone marrow, resulting in the loss of a great number of white blood cells. Other people who could benefit from a substance that stimulates bone marrow cells are the millions of people with depressed immune systems due to aging, stress, or chronic disease.

To understand how melatonin stimulates bone marrow cells is to gain insight into the complexity and interdependence of the immune system. Essentially, melatonin functions as the first runner in a well-trained relay team. To set the race in motion, melatonin links with its receptor on the T-helper cell. The T-helper cell is the next team player, producing more of the IL-4-like factor. This factor then takes the baton and stimulates the production of a substance called granulocyte-macrophage colony-stimulating factor, which (mercifully) is referred to as GM-CSF. GM-CSF, the last runner in the team, sends a stimulatory message to stem cells located in the bone marrow.[19] The net effect of this cooperative venture is that you have a new bounty of white blood cells to help protect you from disease.

Although it is now possible to stimulate bone marrow cells by giving patients a synthetic version of GM-CSF, the synthetic compound is expensive and can cause side effects such as fever and nausea. Melatonin is nontoxic, inexpensive, and free of negative side effects, and it may be just as effective.

CHAPTER 5

▼

NEW HOPE FOR AIDS PATIENTS

The people who may most urgently need melatonin's life-giving actions are those with acquired immunodeficiency syndrome, or AIDS. In the United States, one million people are believed to be infected with the human immunodeficiency virus (HIV), the virus that causes AIDS. Worldwide, the number may be as high as 16 million. Meanwhile, the death toll is mounting. AIDS is now the *leading* cause of death in Americans between the ages of 25 and 44.

HIV may be one of the most cunning diseases to assault the human body. The virus insinuates itself into the very immune cells that are supposed to hold it in check. Once inside, it commandeers the internal machinery of the cell to make copies of itself. It does this by inserting a self-serving set of instructions into the cell's DNA. When decoded, the message reads, "Make more of me." The cell is programmed to oblige. In effect, the virus converts the immune cell into a factory that churns out enemy weapons, flooding the body with viral particles.

Typically, a person infected with HIV is free of symptoms for a number of years. Originally, it was thought that the virus was lying dormant or was replicating at a slow rate. When a person began having symptoms, it was believed to be a sign that the virus had become more active.

Data published in 1995 reveals a strikingly different view of the disease. Researchers now believe that the virus replicates at a furious pace from the moment of infection, churning out as many as 2 billion new viral particles each day.[1] The reason that the patient remains symptom free for some time is that the immune system is creating new cells at an equally impressive rate. This silent invisible battle rages for years. As long as the two forces are of comparable strength, the patient has few symptoms, thus giving the false impression that the virus is dormant.

A healthy person might be able to fend off the virus indefinitely if not for one complication—HIV is not a fixed target. The virus mutates continuously, forcing the body to deal with an ever-changing enemy. Just when the immune system has gotten a clear fix on the virus and has produced millions of tailor-made antibodies, the body is swarming with new mutant viruses. It takes the immune system a number of days to craft antibodies to attack these mutant clones. In the meantime the virus multiplies with impunity.[2]

The stronger a person's immune system, the longer he or she can fight off the mutant clones. But ultimately HIV—with its ceaseless, shifting, diabolical attack—gains the upper hand. As it does, the number of healthy immune cells plummets, and the body becomes easy prey to cancer, bacteria, parasites, protozoa, fungi, and other deadly viruses. It's not HIV itself that is the ultimate cause of death but the opportunistic diseases that survive and thrive because of the collapse of the body's immune system.

GIVING THE IMMUNE SYSTEM AN EDGE

The awareness that the immune system puts out a prodigious effort to defeat HIV has prompted researchers to find new ways to help it do its job. Perhaps, researchers speculate, a significant increase in immune strength would allow the body to triumph over the virus—or at least prolong the period of relative good health. A promising strategy is to find out how the body stimulates the production of immune cells and then try to duplicate that process. The body accomplishes this feat, researchers have learned, by secreting cytokines. These cytokines stimulate the immune cells to divide at a faster rate. Through expensive and sophisticated technology, researchers have been able to synthesize one of the key cytokines, interleukin-2. A recent clinical trial has shown that when synthetic IL-2 is injected into AIDS patients, their bodies produce a great deal more CD4 or T-helper cells, key cells that are lost as the disease progresses.[3]

One problem with this new immunotherapy is that IL-2 can be quite toxic, which introduces a new set of problems. A safer and perhaps equally effective strategy may be to give patients melatonin instead. As we saw in Chapter 4, a group of cancer patients who were given 10 milligrams of melatonin each night for a period of a month had an average 51 percent increase in their level of IL-2.[4] Says Maestroni, "When you give IL-2 to patients, you get a toxic response. When you give melatonin, you get more IL-2."

HOW DOES MELATONIN HELP SLOW THE PROGRESSION OF HIV?

There are three reasons that melatonin shows promise as an adjunct therapy for people with AIDS:
1. It modulates the immune system.
2. It is a potent antioxidant.
3. It may slow the replication of the HIV virus.

A NEW WEAPON FOR THE ARSENAL

Not only does melatonin increase IL-2, it stimulates the production of a number of other immune components known to be deficient in people infected with HIV, including natural killer cells, interferon-gamma, IL-4, IL-10, eosinophils, and red blood cells.[5] [6]

Interestingly, melatonin also *inhibits* the production of certain immune components, which paradoxically could prove just as beneficial for people with HIV. It is quite common for AIDS patients to have an inflammatory disease, caused in part by an abundance of leukotrienes, substances that contribute to the inflammatory response.[7] (In excess, leukotrienes can add to the discomfort of other conditions such as arthritis, asthma, and various allergic reactions.) We have recently learned that melatonin inhibits their production. A 1995 experiment revealed that melatonin causes a fivefold reduction in the production of leukotrienes.[8] According to a recent article in *Virus Research*, inhibitors of leukotrienes are "promising anti-HIV compounds."[9]

There are additional ways that melatonin modifies the immune system that might be beneficial in the treatment of HIV. These ways are listed in the chart on pages 73 to 77. As you will see, the chart has not been composed with the average lay person in mind. It is intended for use by medical professionals and by the many people with HIV who, in their valiant efforts to stay well, have become as knowledgeable about the immune system as some physicians.

HOW FREE RADICALS CONTRIBUTE TO AIDS

Not only does melatonin enhance the immune system, it may also help defeat HIV by getting rid of free radicals. AIDS researchers have discovered that free radicals play a significant role in the progression of the disease. They discovered this fact while in the process of solving a puzzle: Some of the immune cells that were being destroyed in the course of HIV were not infected with the virus. If the virus wasn't killing them, what was?

The virus-free immune cells were being damaged by free radicals, the researchers found out. One of the weapons that the immune system uses to attack HIV is a substance called tumor necrosis factor, or TNF, which produces free radicals. As the virus multiplies, the immune system, like a sorcerer's misguided apprentice, produces ever more TNF, which results in ever more free radicals. Eventually, so many free radicals are created that healthy immune cells become vulnerable to damage.

At first, the healthy immune cells are able to protect themselves from this friendly fire by drawing on their abundant supply of glutathione, one of the body's most important antioxidants. But eventually the supply of glutathione becomes depleted, and the free radicals cause extensive damage. When an immune cell becomes damaged beyond repair, the DNA molecule sends it a message to self-destruct—a quality-control measure designed to keep abnormal cells from becoming malignant. Unfortunately, the loss of these immune cells further erodes the body's defenses.

Given this new insight into the mechanics of HIV, researchers became interested in developing antioxidant therapies and are now beginning to give them to AIDS patients. One of the compounds being tested is N-acetylcysteine, or NAC, a compound that helps form glutathione. (NAC is also taken by many HIV-positive people outside clinical trials.) The hope is that taking NAC will increase the body's supply of glutathione, allowing more T cells to survive.

It's a sound theory, but NAC may not be the best antioxidant for the job. Melatonin appears to be more effective at protecting cells from free-radical damage than any known antioxidant, be it glutathione, beta carotene, or vitamin E.[10] Furthermore, melatonin stimulates the action of the related antioxidant glutathione peroxidase, which has also been deemed useful in the fight against AIDS.[11]

MELATONIN MAY INHIBIT VIRAL REPLICATION

A third reason that melatonin may help defeat AIDS is that it may slow the replication of the virus itself. This finding also emerged from our laboratory. In an animal experiment conducted in 1995, my colleagues and I found that melatonin inhibits a substance called nuclear factor kappa-B (NF-κB).[12] This substance is an essential link in the chain of events that leads to the cloning of HIV. When NF-κB is inhibited, the virus divides more slowly. One reason we decided to explore a possible link between NF-κB and melatonin is that we learned that the actions of NF-κB are reduced by as much as 23 percent during the night—precisely when melatonin is present in the highest concentration. Could melatonin be inhibiting NF-κB? By injecting rats with melatonin during the daytime, we found the answer. The melatonin injections reduced the binding activity of NF-κB by 43 percent, suggesting that melatonin may be able to inhibit the rate of division of HIV.

A PILOT AIDS STUDY

Georges Maestroni and his colleagues, pioneers in the field of melatonin immunotherapy, were the first to suggest that melatonin might be of immense value to AIDS patients. In 1987 they tested their theory by giving melatonin to eleven HIV-infected individuals. (Two of these patients were asymptomatic, and the remainder had advanced cases of AIDS.[13]) The therapy was inexpensive, nontoxic, and easy to administer: At seven o'clock each evening, each patient took a 20-milligram tablet of melatonin. The only side effect they reported was a better night's sleep.

To see what effect melatonin was having on the disease, the researchers gave the patients blood tests at regular intervals. At the end of fourteen days of treatment, they found that the three patients who had the most advanced cases of AIDS had a 232 percent increase in peripheral blood mononuclear cells, or PBMC. After a month of treatment, the patients overall had a 35 percent increase in T-helper cells (CD4 cells), a 57 percent increase in natural killer cells, and a 76 percent increase in null cells (a type of lymphocyte).[14] This response is all the more remarkable given that melatonin is a natural, nontoxic substance.

▶ MELATONIN COMBATS WASTING SYNDROME

Melatonin benefited the AIDS patients in other ways as well. Those who were the most debilitated by the disease were suffering from wasting syndrome, a combination of lethargy and weight loss. There are a number of ways to treat wasting syndrome, but most of them are prohibitively expensive. Regular injections of growth hormone, for example, can restore patients' appetites, but this treatment costs as much as a thousand dollars per week.[15] Another remedy, called total parenteral nutrition, which involves giving patients highly concentrated nutrients through a catheter, is even more expensive. Lacking the necessary finances, some patients opt for a cheaper and less sanctioned appetite stimulant—smoking marijuana or taking tablets containing THC, the active ingredient in marijuana.[16]

Melatonin may prove to be an effective, inexpensive—and legal—treatment for wasting syndrome. A number of patients in Maestroni's study gained a significant amount of weight and had a noticeable improvement in their overall status.[17]

▶ SUGGESTED TREATMENT PROTOCOL

The number of patients enrolled in Maestroni's pilot study was small, and the disease in many of them was at an advanced stage—within weeks of starting the treatment, two patients died and a third developed dementia and had to be institutionalized. Therefore, no definitive conclusions can be drawn from the study. But Maestroni believes that melatonin demonstrated enough promise in the study to justify a larger clinical trial.

The pilot study also gave Maestroni a vital piece of information about treatment protocol. The patients showed the greatest response to melatonin, he found, after two or three weeks of treatment, after which time the number of their immune cells began to decline. He believes that if patients had a one-week washout period after every three or four weeks of treatment, their immune response would remain at a consistently higher level.

MELATONIN—AN IDEAL SLEEP MEDICATION FOR AIDS PATIENTS

Many AIDS patients suffer from insomnia. (Sleep medications account for 43 percent of the psychoactive drugs prescribed for this particular group of patients.[18]) Insomnia may seem a minor complaint when compared with the other problems caused by the disease, but it erodes one's quality of life and impairs the ability to recuperate and fight off disease.

The drugs commonly prescribed for sleep, benzodiazepines, help AIDS patients fall asleep, but they may also *diminish* their immune response. Some benzodiazepines can interfere with the immune system by inhibiting the body's production of melatonin. (For example, a 2-milligram dose of alprazolam taken in the evening can reduce a person's melatonin levels throughout the night.[19]) Another problem with traditional sleep medications is that most of them interfere with deep sleep. Taking benzodiazepines for weeks at a time can abolish deep sleep altogether.[20] Deep sleep is vital for people with chronic diseases because the immune system appears to be most active during this particular stage of the sleep cycle. Deep sleep may be especially beneficial for AIDS patients with wasting syndrome because the body produces most of its growth hormone during this critical stage. (Growth hormone stimulates the appetite and helps preserve body mass.)

Melatonin may be an ideal sleep aid for AIDS patients. As we will see in more detail in Chapter 8, melatonin promotes a deep and restful sleep, allowing the body to use the nighttime as it was intended—as a much-needed time of rest and repair.

MELATONIN PLUS AZT (ZDV)

Although melatonin may offer AIDS patients a banquet of benefits, the hormone alone will not defeat the disease once it has reached an advanced stage. But if people infected with HIV take melatonin during the initial stages of the disease, and/or in conjunction with other substances, the hormone may cause a significant slowing of the disease.

One possibility worth exploring is to combine melatonin with AZT (azidothymidine, also known as Zidovudine or ZDV). AZT is a widely prescribed drug that slows the progression of HIV infection, decreases the incidence of opportunistic infections, and may prolong survival. But AZT can cause nausea, vomiting, insomnia, headaches, and fatigue. Furthermore, it is toxic to bone marrow, resulting in a significant reduction in both white and red blood cells. To counteract this toxicity, some patients on AZT have been given substances called colony-stimulating factors. But colony-stimulating factors are expensive to administer and produce negative side effects of their own.

Melatonin may be the better alternative. Maestroni has shown that melatonin increases production of the body's *own* colony-stimulating factor—granulocyte-macrophage colony-stimulating factor, or GM-CSF.[21]

This strategy has already helped at least one AIDS patient, whose case Maestroni described to me while I was visiting him in his new laboratory in Locarno. An American named Douglas, the son of a well-known immunologist, had an advanced case of AIDS. The father heard about Maestroni's work with melatonin and suggested that Douglas seek him out at his clinic in Switzerland. When Douglas arrived in Switzerland, he was very ill and was thought to have but a few months to live. One of his many problems was that he was suffering from the side effects of AZT. So toxic was the drug to his bone marrow that he was being given blood transfusions every two weeks. At Maestroni's suggestion, Douglas began taking 20 milligrams of melatonin at bedtime. Immediately, he was able to go six weeks between blood transfusions instead of his customary two.[22] As Maestroni had predicted, melatonin buffered the toxicity of AZT, a protective action that since has been observed in cancer patients who take melatonin along with chemotherapy.[23]

Melatonin did more for Douglas than counteract the toxicity of AZT, however. His mood and energy level improved, and he put on weight. After a few months, he flew back home to the United States. Still, melatonin was not able to save his life, and he died eighteen months later.

Maestroni believes the hormone will prove most beneficial when taken at a much earlier stage of the disease. "Melatonin's main mode of action is to link with the CD4+ cell," he explains. "If that cell population is already decimated, melatonin has little to work with. In the later stages, it can help diminish the toxicity of other drugs and may improve the overall quality of life, but it won't be able to stave off the disease."

MELATONIN PLUS INTERLEUKIN-2

In 1993, Maestroni and Conti suggested a further use for melatonin in the treatment of HIV: combining it with IL-2. This combination immunotherapy, they had found, was more effective in treating cancer in animals than either substance alone. They had reason to believe the novel therapy might prove superior for treating HIV as well.[24]

To test this possibility, Maestroni and Conti joined with Paolo Lissoni, a neuroimmunologist from San Gerardo Hospital in Monza, Italy. Lissoni is a pioneer in alternative treatments. For example, he encourages his cancer patients to reduce their stress by practicing yoga and meditation, techniques yet to be sanctioned in most medical schools.

Lissoni has ambitious goals. His vision is to develop nontoxic, effective immunotherapies for diseases now regarded as untreatable, including AIDS and advanced metastatic cancer. His quest has led him to melatonin. The findings that Maestroni and Conti produce in the lab, Lissoni applies to humans. So far, he has administered melatonin to more than 350 patients in clinical trials.

Lissoni and his colleagues at San Gerardo Hospital began giving AIDS patients the IL-2 plus melatonin therapy.

Their protocol was simple: Every evening, the patients were given a low-dose injection of IL-2 and a 20-milligram tablet of melatonin.[25] (The medication was given in the evening because studies had shown both substances to be more effective when administered then.)

The study lasted for one month. On average, the patients showed a significant increase in levels of natural killer cells and activated T cells, as well as an improvement in the ratio of T-helper to suppresser T cells, a factor that is regarded as an indicator of the progression of the disease.[26] The treatment did not increase viral replication, a problem that has been observed in some forms of immunotherapy.

THE NEED FOR LARGER AND MORE COMPREHENSIVE STUDIES

Given melatonin's lack of toxicity, its ability to stimulate so many diverse elements of the immune system, its talent for destroying free radicals, and its potential to slow the replication of HIV, a large-scale melatonin AIDS trial is needed immediately. Maestroni made such a plea in a 1993 article. He wrote:

> Chronic, periodic [three weeks on and one week off] melatonin treatment should be evaluated for its potential benefit in asymptomatic, HIV-positive individuals. Here one would consider that both HIV and melatonin seem to have the same target, i.e., $CD4^+$ T lymphocytes, and thus melatonin might be eventually helpful before the development of AIDS, i.e., in presence of a normal or sustained concentration of $CD4^+$ T lymphocytes. These large and long-term studies should be multi-centered and possibly supported by pharmaceutical concerns or by international organizations.[27]

Regrettably, as this book goes to press, Maestroni's plea has yet to be answered. The fact that melatonin is a natural substance and cannot be patented has prevented pharmaceutical companies from investing the millions of dollars that would be needed to conduct such a trial. Meanwhile, government health agencies have yet to show interest. Because of this lack of response, an unknown number of AIDS patients have begun taking melatonin on their own, entering into an unfunded, unsupervised experiment that may confer individual benefits to them but yield little in the way of useful data. Since melatonin seems tailor-made to take on HIV, theirs is an understandable course of action. I wish them well.

HOW MELATONIN MIGHT HELP PEOPLE WITH HIV

MELATONIN'S ACTIONS	BENEFICIAL EFFECTS
Lymphocytes	
Restores T-helper cell activity[28]	• Increases resistance to pathogens and tumors[29]
Stimulates IL-2[30]	• IL-2 increases production of T-helper cells. Adding melatonin to an IL-2 treatment program may allow a lower dose of IL-2 to be used without compromising treatment.[31]
Stimulates IFN-gamma[32]	IFM-gamma: • With TNF alpha inhibits hematopoiesis.[33] • Is hypothesized to play key role with Rifabutin and in treatment of MAC infections.[34] • Protects primary monocytes against infection with HIV-1.[35] • Blocks HIV-1 infection of HT-29-A7 cells.[36] • Increases cytotoxic effect of AZT.[37]

Stimulates an IL-4-like factor[38]

IL-4:
- Induces a latent stage in viral replication.[39]
- With IL-13, increases IL-1 receptor antagonist secretion by macrophages.[40]
- With IL-13 protects bronchoalveolar macrophages from infection.[41]
- Regulates both normal and pathological hematopoiesis.[42]

Stimulates GM-CSF[43]

GM-CSF:
- Modulates virus replication in monocytes/macrophages.[44]
- Prevents HIV-1 replication in vitro.[45]
- Improves white and red blood cell counts in AIDS patients.[46]
- Protects bone marrow from the toxic effects of INF-alpha and AZT.[47]

Stimulates natural killer cells[48]

- Impaired NK cell function may promote multidrug resistance.[49]
- A decrease in NK-cell function is related to progression of HIV infection.[50]
- CD16+ NK cells decrease in all stages of HIV infection.[51]

Increases null cells[52]	Null cells participate in immunoglobulin synthesis in B cells.[53]
Stimulates salivary IgA[54]	AIDS patients have low levels of salivary IgA.[55] Salivary IgA protects against upper respiratory infections.
Macrophages	
Reduces neopterin[56]	HIV-1 infection is accompanied by increased neopterin concentrations; higher neopterin levels predict more rapid disease progression.[57]
Increases eosinophils[58]	Increase in eosinophil cell count and their activation may be important in AIDS.[59]
Platelets	
Increases platelets	Many AIDS patients have a deficiency of platelets, which can lead to hemorrhage.[60]

Antioxidants

Has potent antioxidant properties[61]	• Reduced antioxidant levels are risk factors for onset and development of AIDS.[62 63 64] • Some antioxidants block role of NF-κB in HIV activation.[65] • Beta carotene stimulates immune system in HIV-infected patients.[66] • Antioxidants may prevent the free-radical-mediated demise of uninfected T cells.[67]
Stimulates glutathione peroxidase (Gpx)[68]	Gpx: • Decreases NF-κB activation by H_2O_2. • Induces a protective effect against cell activation by TNF-α. • Increased Gpx in latently infected T lymphocytes protects against cytotoxic and reactivating effects of hydrogen peroxide.

Other Properties

Represses 5-lipoxygenase[69]	• Results in fewer leukotrienes, which may help reduce the inflammatory response seen in many AIDS patients.

Combats wasting syndrome[70]	• AIDS patients who have taken melatonin have gained weight and shown an improved quality of life.
Stimulates growth hormone[71]	• Growth hormone is effective in treating wasting syndrome.
Enhances sleep[72]	• A majority of AIDS patients have sleep difficulties. Melatonin is a safe and natural sleep aid that does not disrupt normal sleep patterns.

CHAPTER 6

▼

TAMING THE SAVAGE CELL

Dora L., 70, lives in Montreal. She is an avid bridge player and health enthusiast. She is also a cancer survivor. When she was diagnosed with carcinoma of the thyroid in 1987, her thyroid was removed. By 1989, the cancer had spread to nearby lymph nodes; these, too, were removed. In the process of removing one of the nodes, the surgeon may have nicked a nerve, paralyzing Dora's right vocal cord. To this day, she speaks in a hoarse whisper.

Following this particular surgery, Dora's endocrinologist suggested that she undergo radiation therapy to keep the cancer from spreading any further. Dora was not comfortable with the idea of radiation, but, she says, "I didn't know what else to do." She underwent thirty sessions of intense radiation, which caused sores in her mouth and throat and on various parts of her head. "My earlobes turned black," she recalls, "and I was always choking. The symptoms got worse as the treatment progressed. I still have problems. I have all kind of sores in my mouth and neck, my mouth especially."

And still the cancer came back. In 1993 a body scan showed that she had a tumor three and a half centimeters long on her right lung. Her pulmonary specialist wanted to operate so he could get a close look at the extent of the metastases. If necessary, he would remove the lung. This time Dora balked. Her left lung had collapsed during heart surgery ten years earlier, and she was afraid that if they removed her right lung, her remaining lung would collapse again. Her fear was that she "would die on the operating table with none of my family around me."

Dora didn't want the surgery, but she wasn't ready to die either. She decided to consult a local physician, Dr. Roman Rozencweig, who was interested in alternative medicine. Take melatonin, Rozencweig advised her. "What is this melatonin?" she asked him. "I've never heard about it." Rozencweig told her all he knew about the hormone. After deliberating, Dora decided to follow his advice and take 6 milligrams each evening.

In a matter of months, Dora felt considerably better. "I had more energy. I began walking for an hour a day." She also joined a cancer group called Hope and Cope and gained a great deal of support from other cancer survivors. In turn, she told them about melatonin. "I even brought a bottle to show them," she says. "I told them that my doctor had advised me to take it." The other members of the group were excited about melatonin, and many of them later asked their own doctors if they should take it. Says Dora, "None of their doctors knew anything about melatonin, so they would not recommend it. I was the only one who would take it."

In the spring of 1995, Dora went to her oncologist for a periodic check-up. To her delight, she learned that the growth in her lung had shrunk by more than a centimeter and that there appeared to be no other metastases. She shared the good news with her support group at the next meeting—"at least with those who were still alive," she adds. "By this time, some of the women who joined when I did were no longer there."

Dora's story illustrates a fundamental aspect of medical ethics: Before most doctors will prescribe any therapy—especially a therapy for a life-threatening disease such as cancer—they must be convinced that it is both safe and effective. What convinces them is neither rave reviews from patients nor glowing articles in health magazines but large-scale human studies. Without such studies, they have no way to know if a given treatment is a fad or a truly effective therapy. This is especially true when it comes to treating cancer, an area of medicine in which dozens of substances, from shark cartilage to Kombuchu mushrooms, are touted as "natural miracle" cures. It would be unethical for a doctor to prescribe any of these products without convincing scientific proof.

I applaud the fact that the medical profession demands rigorous evidence. If, God forbid, my wife had cancer, I would not want her to take unproven pills and potions recommended by friends or selected at random from the shelves of a health-food store. Instead, I would hope she would place herself in the hands of a highly trained oncologist who would recommend a treatment plan that had been proven to be equal or superior to all other treatments. But I would also encourage her to select a physician who had a holistic philosophy of healing and who viewed her not as a host for a tumor but as a living, breathing human being with opinions, thoughts, feelings, a distinct medical history, and a unique lifestyle. I would want this physician to be cognizant of the fact that certain foods and food supplements have *proven* healing properties. But my most ardent wish would be that this doctor agree with us that a therapy that stimulates the body's natural healing process is superior to one that compromises it with toxins, radiation, or surgery—*provided that the therapy has been proven to be both safe and effective*.

Using these criteria, this chapter will answer the following questions: (1) What has been proven about melatonin's ability to prevent and/or treat cancer? (2) How reliable are the studies? (3) What is melatonin's potential role in the prevention and treatment of cancer?

EARLY PIONEERS

It has been known for more than a century that some unknown substance manufactured by the pineal gland blocks cancer growth in both animals and humans. In the late 1800s and early 1900s, a number of medical doctors acted on this knowledge and began giving ground-up pineal extracts to cancer patients. Reports of a number of partial and even complete responses are sprinkled throughout the literature.

To my knowledge, the first time that melatonin in a purified form was given to cancer patients was in 1963, just five years after the hormone had been isolated and identified. A Welsh physician named Kenneth Starr gave intravenous infusions of melatonin to a young man who had a tumor in his leg that had spread to lymph nodes in his groin and neck. Starr reports that the "melatonin infusion resulted in the disappearance of the masses within ten days."[1]

Another one of Starr's "miracle cures" was a sixteen-year-old boy with a tumor (osteogenic sarcoma) on his shinbone. Starr writes:

> The patient was admitted for amputation but was given an infusion of melatonin while awaiting radiotherapy and healing of the biopsy wound. The clinical and biochemical response was evident in the second week. Radiotherapy was begun, but in the second month suspicious shadows appeared in the lung fields, considered to be metastases. By the end of the fourth month these had disappeared, and the lung fields have remained clear. The stiff, painful knee has improved, and he can now run, jump, and ride a horse.

Isolated cases such as these carry little weight in the medical community, especially if the researcher is not well known and shares few of his procedural details. But Starr's pioneering efforts served a useful purpose nonetheless: They brought melatonin to the attention of a number of cancer researchers, who then began a more systematic investigation.

For almost two decades progress was slow as researchers struggled to understand the complexities of the molecule, and for the most part the research was limited to animal studies. But some of these animal studies were filled with promise. One of the more compelling studies was conducted by an American researcher named Lawrence Tamarkin. In 1980, Tamarkin injected a group of rats with a carcinogen called DMBA, which stimulates the growth of breast tumors.[2] (DMBA-induced mammary tumors are believed to closely resemble human breast cancer.) To see if melatonin offered any protective effect, he gave some of the rats a daily dose of the hormone as well. At the end of ninety days, 50 percent of the rats that were not treated with melatonin had breast tumors compared with *none* of the melatonin-treated animals. At this point in the study, Tamarkin stopped giving melatonin to the melatonin-treatment group, and eventually 20 percent of those rats developed mammary tumors as well.[3]

BREAST CANCER

Animal studies such as Tamarkin's prompted researchers to explore melatonin's effects on human cancer cells. One of the leaders in the field is my former student David Blask, M.D., Ph.D., now at the Mary Imogene Bassett Research Institute in Cooperstown, New York. In a study published in 1986, Blask decided to see if melatonin could inhibit the growth of a virulent strain of human breast cancer cells known as MCF-7 cells. (Like most cancer cells used in medical research, these cells are clones of tumor cells removed from an actual patient and kept alive in a medium that fosters growth. Such cells are referred to as "cancer cell lines" and are given a specific code name. Researchers all over the world can use clones of the very same cells, making it easier to compare results.)

Assisted by post-doctoral student Steven Hill, Blask divided the breast cancer cells into two groups. Their plan was to add melatonin to one of the batches of cells. If melatonin had an inhibitory effect, those cells should divide at a slower rate than the untreated batch. Not knowing how much melatonin to add, Blask and Hill added a relatively large amount. In Blask's own words, "like any good chemists we dumped in a bunch of melatonin." They wanted to make sure that any potential effect would be perceptible. But even though the cells were exposed to a hundred times more melatonin than is present in the human bloodstream, they continued to thrive.

The researchers repeated the experiment a number of times and came up with the same results: There was no difference in the rate of growth between the cells that were growing with and without melatonin.

Blask and Hill were about to conclude that melatonin had no effect on the cells, when it dawned on Blask that

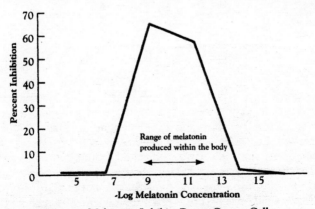

Figure 9. Melatonin Inhibits Breast Cancer Cells

they might be using *too much* melatonin. "Maybe less is more," he suggested to Hill. "The body produces so little of it, maybe it works best in small quantities." They went back to the lab and repeated the experiment, using much smaller amounts of the hormone. To their surprise, a mere smattering of melatonin blocked the growth of the breast cancer cells by 75 percent. This finding was unexpected since virtually all anticancer compounds are most effective in high concentrations. Melatonin apparently works the other way around.

Intrigued, Blask and Hill went on to see if they could determine the most effective concentration of melatonin. This phase of the study produced an even more remarkable finding: Melatonin had the greatest effect in a very particular range—a range that happens to be the amount of melatonin present in the human body. Concentrations above and below that amount had no effect on the cells.[4] "We were stunned," Blask says. "We had a phenomenon we couldn't explain. It was easy to understand why very small concentrations of melatonin had no effect. But why were high amounts ineffective? All that we knew was that, for some reason, a woman's body produces *precisely* the amount of melatonin required to slow the growth of these breast cancer cells. The body knew something that we didn't."

▶ MIMICKING THE BODY'S OWN PLAN

Not until eight years later did anyone think to take Blask and Hill's experiment to the next logical step. A Spanish researcher named Samuel Cos, who had spent time working in Blask's lab, asked himself what no one else had bothered to ask: Why had Blask and Hill incubated the breast cancer cells in a constant amount of melatonin when the body produces the hormone in a distinct circadian fashion—high at night and low during the day? What would happen in a test-tube experiment that mimicked this rhythm?

Cos obtained clones of the same breast cancer cells used by Blask and Hill. After dividing them into a number of different groups, he incubated each group in a different manner. Some he incubated continuously in the amount of melatonin the body produces at night, others in daytime concentrations. Still others were incubated in alternating concentrations—high for twelve hours and then low for twelve hours—replicating the body's circadian cycle. As Cos had surmised, the cancer cells that showed the least growth were the ones incubated in the alternating concentrations.[5] Once again, mimicking the body's own strategy had produced the best results.

These test-tube experiments strongly suggest that melatonin is part of a woman's built-in defense against breast cancer. When melatonin is present in the concentrations produced by the body and in accordance with its circadian rhythm, it is a potent anticancer agent. One of melatonin's roles may be to inhibit the growth of errant breast cancer cells, making them easier for immune cells to tackle.

This theory may help explain why the risk of breast cancer increases with age. Of all the known risk factors for breast cancer—early menstruation, late menopause, eating a high-fat diet, drinking alcohol, having no children, having the first child late in life, not breast-feeding, having a close relative with breast cancer, advancing age—the one that best predicts whether a woman will get breast cancer is her age. In fact, two-thirds of all women with breast cancer have no known risk factors *other* than advancing age.

It has been well documented that as women age, they produce less melatonin. Perhaps older women no longer produce enough of the hormone to keep random breast cancer cells in check, increasing the chances that the cells will develop into full-blown tumors.

▶ CAN MELATONIN HELP *PREVENT*
   BREAST CANCER?

If declining levels of melatonin do indeed result in an increased risk of breast cancer—and I must emphasize that it is just a theory—we may well ask whether taking melatonin supplements will reduce the risk. No one knows. The answer must come from a large, long-term clinical trial, similar to the ongoing breast cancer prevention study involving the anti-estrogen drug tamoxifen.

Regrettably, no one is conducting such a study; nor to my knowledge is one being planned. According to Amy Langer, executive director of the National Alliance of Breast Cancer Organizations, this omission is a major failing of current breast cancer research. "Cancer scientists have done a lot of research on treating cancer, but very little on prevention. We need a real breakthrough in prevention. Unfortunately, researchers in the United States have been slow to investigate the body's own mechanisms."[6]

In the meantime, the best we can do is glean what insight we can from other data. One potential source of information is the ongoing clinical trial of the B-Oval pill, a novel contraceptive that contains 75 milligrams of melatonin. Fourteen hundred women in Holland have been taking the B-Oval pill for over four years. As in any clinical trial, the health of the women is being closely monitored, including their incidence of breast cancer. It will be several years before the study is concluded. Unfortunately, there may be too few women enrolled in the study to provide statistically significant data about melatonin's effects on breast cancer.

Michael Cohen, M.D., Ph.D., director of Applied Medical Research Ltd. and the developer of the B-Oval pill, is keenly interested in finding a preventive treatment for breast cancer. In 1978, years before the conclusive evidence that melatonin inhibits breast cancer cells, Cohen published an article in *Lancet* suggesting that melatonin may reduce the risk of breast cancer by inhibiting the reproductive hormones, especially estrogen.[7]

He backs up this contention with an intriguing theory. Humans have a much higher incidence of breast cancer than other mammals. This difference may be due to the fact that we are no longer seasonal breeders, Cohen contends. A woman's breasts are exposed all year long to the stimulatory effects of estrogen and other reproductive hormones—substances known to promote the growth of breast cancer cells. Melatonin has an inhibitory effect on many reproductive hormones, including estrogen. Women who have low levels of melatonin—whether from aging, environmental factors, or hereditary factors—may be at even greater risk for breast cancer, he believes.

Cohen has launched a study whose sole purpose is to

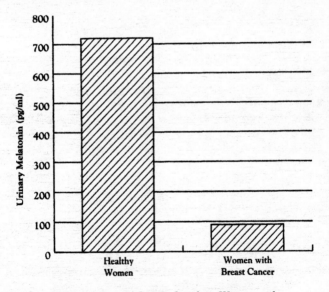

Figure 10. Low Melatonin Levels in Women with Breast Cancer

In one study there was a marked difference in nocturnal melatonin levels between women with and without breast cancer.

explore melatonin's effects on breast cancer. In this study, women who are planning to have breast-reduction surgery are randomly selected to take either the B-Oval pill or a birth control pill that does not include melatonin. A year later, they have their surgery, and the excised breast tissue is examined closely to determine the effect of the two different preparations. This project is nearing completion and may shed some light on melatonin's effects on human breast tissue.[8] Langer says, "I believe the science behind Cohen's theory is very sound. Melatonin has encouraging potential for breast cancer prevention and treatment."[9]

▶ MELATONIN AS A THERAPY
   FOR BREAST CANCER

Does melatonin hold any promise for *treating* breast cancer? Each year, approximately 182,000 American women are diagnosed with the disease.[10] If melatonin can slow the growth of breast cancer cells in test tubes, will it also reduce tumor growth in women?

To date, no researcher has produced strong evidence that melatonin alone will cure any kind of advanced cancer, including breast cancer. *But there is growing evidence that when melatonin is combined with other therapies, whether traditional or investigational, the patients live longer and fare better.*

One promising new therapy combines melatonin with tamoxifen. Tamoxifen is the most widely used oncology agent in the world, but like all anticancer drugs, it has its limitations. Some breast cancer cell types do not respond to it, while others respond for only a limited time. Moreover, even if tamoxifen inhibits breast cancer, it may increase patients' risk of uterine and other cancers. Thus, combining melatonin with tamoxifen could have two significant benefits: lowering the required dose of tamoxifen and improving the drug's effectiveness. The net effect may be a greater inhibition of tumor growth and fewer negative side effects.

The originator of this theory is David Blask. Melatonin and tamoxifen, he observed, perform a number of similar actions, including blocking estrogen from stimulating the growth of breast cancer cells.[11] A therapy combining the two substances, he reasoned, might be more effective than either one used in isolation. As an initial test of the theory, he and two colleagues, Sean Wilson and Athena Lemus-Wilson, cultured human breast cancer cells in a dilute concentration of melatonin for twenty-four hours. Then they added tamoxifen. To their wonderment, pretreating the cells with melatonin amplified the potency of tamoxifen one hundred times![12]

▶ MELATONIN AND TAMOXIFEN IN COMBINATION

The import of this finding was recognized immediately by Paolo Lissoni, the immunologist who conducted the melatonin plus IL-2 AIDS study. Working with a group of colleagues from San Gerardo Hospital, he gave melatonin along with tamoxifen to fourteen women with advanced metastatic breast cancer who were not responding to any other treatment. All of the women had been treated with tamoxifen before joining the study and had either failed to respond to the drug or had stopped responding after a time.

The women were given both melatonin and tamoxifen in tablet form—20 milligrams of tamoxifen at noon and 20 milligrams of melatonin in the evening. None of them experienced significant toxic side effects. "On the contrary," Lissoni reported in a 1995 article in *The British Journal of Cancer*, "most patients experienced a relief of anxiety; moreover, a relief of depressant symptoms occurred in three patients. Finally, two other patients . . . had a clear improvement in their quality of life."[13]

The effect of the therapy on the breast tumors themselves was just as encouraging. Four of the fourteen women had a 50 percent or greater reduction in the size of their tumors. Eight additional women showed no further progression in tumor size. Only two women failed to respond to the treatment. These results are all the more impressive given the fact that the therapy *improved* the quality of the women's lives. As most cancer patients will attest, traditional cancer therapy can be a tremendous ordeal, causing nausea, fatigue, depression, and anxiety. Some people are so wary of these negative side effects that they elect not to receive treatment at all.

Lissoni is now planning a randomized study to compare the results of the combination therapy with tamoxifen alone. If he and others can replicate the findings from his pilot study in larger controlled studies, women may one day have less reason to fear a diagnosis of breast cancer.[14]

Meanwhile, back in the United States, efforts to develop a melatonin-tamoxifen therapy are progressing more slowly, partly due to the stricter standards imposed by the FDA and partly because of a lack of interest on the part of funding agencies. As a result, Blask has been unable to get the necessary approval and funding to test his therapy on humans.

He has gotten encouraging results, however, from a just completed animal study. In this study, he implanted a group of mice with human breast cancer cells. When the mice were treated with tamoxifen alone, the growth of their tumors was inhibited by as much as 40 percent early on, but this inhibitory effect decreased in the following weeks. At the conclusion of the study, the tumors were growing just as rapidly in the tamoxifen-treated mice as those in the mice that were given saline alone. Meanwhile, the mice treated with tamoxifen plus melatonin experienced a 60 percent reduction in tumor growth.[15] Blask is hoping that this latest finding, coupled with the results from Lissoni's pilot study, will engender support for a melatonin-tamoxifen clinical trial in the United States.

PROSTATE CANCER

Prostate cancer is the most common form of cancer in men and is second only to lung cancer in mortality rate. Each year, two hundred thousand new cases of prostate cancer are detected in the United States alone, and approximately forty thousand American men die from the disease.[16]

New, as yet unpublished data shows that melatonin inhibits the growth of prostate cancer cells. When David Blask and another group of researchers incubated human prostate cancer cells in melatonin, they got a 50 percent inhibition.[17] The type of cell used in both studies (the DU-145 cell line) does not respond to hormonal treatment. Prostate cancer that cannot be influenced by hormonal manipulation is notoriously difficult to treat. Blask is now making plans to see if melatonin has a similar effect on animals that have been transplanted with these cells.

There are some marked similarities between prostate cancer and breast cancer, which may be why melatonin inhibits both of them. Both types are hormone-dependent for at least the initial stage of their development. (Breast cancer is stimulated by estrogen and prolactin, and prostate cancer is stimulated by testosterone.) Both cancers can be arrested in their early stages, either by surgery or by blocking their respective hormones. After the tumors have metastasized, however, they both become much more difficult to treat. For example, if prostate cancer is treated when it is in a localized state, the five-year survival rate is 70 percent. But once the tumor has spread to another site, the rate drops to 35 percent.[18]

Another similarity between breast cancer and prostate cancer is that some studies have shown that people who have these diseases have unusually low levels of melatonin. Whether the low levels of melatonin contribute to the disease or are a result of it is not yet known.

As far as I know, no one has yet taken this research to the next step and designed a study to give melatonin to

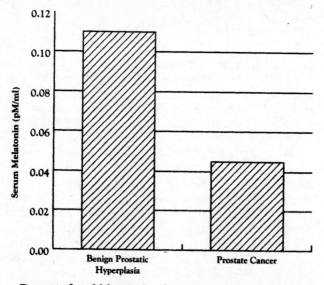

Figure 11. Low Melatonin Levels in Men with Prostate Cancer

In one study, men with prostate cancer produced less melatonin at night than those with enlarged prostate glands (benign prostatic hyperplasia).

prostate cancer patients. But given melatonin's easy availability, a few men with prostate cancer have begun to take the hormone on their own. About a year ago, Steven Rozencweig, a seventy-one-year-old man from Montreal, was diagnosed with prostate cancer. He discovered he had the disease through a routine diagnostic test, the PSA (prostate-specific antigen test). A PSA result of 4 or higher may be a cause for concern; Steven's PSA was 30, indicating a strong likelihood of prostate cancer. A physical examination confirmed the diagnosis. Given Steven's age, however, and the fact that prostate cancer can be slow-growing, his doctor recommended a wait-and-see attitude. In other words, no treatment.

Steven's son happens to be Roman Rozencweig, the Montreal physician who has recommended melatonin to a number of cancer patients (including Dora L., whose story begins this chapter). Following his son's advice, Steven began to take 6 milligrams of melatonin each night. One immediate side effect was that he began to sleep better. But the best news came six months later, when he visited his oncologist for a check-up. The doctor told him that his PSA count had dropped to 13, an indication that the tumor was less active.

Am I suggesting that men with high PSA counts or who have been diagnosed with prostate cancer should take melatonin? Absolutely not. There is far too little data to recommend such a course. Prostate cancer is a deadly disease, and it must be treated by knowledgeable physicians who administer clinically proven therapies. Steven's apparent success with melatonin, however, is one more reason to urge scientists to pursue this promising area of research. It is within the realm of possibility that melatonin might help prevent prostate cancer, slow the progression of the disease, or even, in combination with other treatments, contribute to the long-sought cure.

LUNG CANCER, GASTRIC CANCER, AND LIVER CANCER

Researchers in Europe have been studying melatonin's effects on a variety of other types of tumors, including three of the most deadly—lung cancer, gastric cancer, and liver cancer. So far, more than three hundred patients have participated in these studies.

Paolo Lissoni is conducting these studies as well. His very first melatonin clinical trial for cancer was in 1987 and involved giving injections to nineteen patients. The therapy produced no toxic effects, which is rare for an anticancer treatment. Lissoni notes, "No cardiac, hematological, hepatic, renal or metabolic toxicity was seen in any case during melatonin treatment. Moreover, no undesirable subjective effects were reported."[19] In fact, the patients actually felt *better* while taking melatonin. Many of them felt more relaxed after receiving the injections. All of them slept better. Three of five patients who had lost weight during other cancer therapies regained more than 10 percent of their body weight. Two of five patients suffering from chronic pain were able to reduce their pain medications.

But did the treatment cure them of cancer? The results were modest. Only one patient, a man with pancreatic cancer, had a regression in tumor size. In six of the nineteen patients, tumor growth stopped for a period of time. The remaining patients got steadily worse. But Lissoni was not discouraged by these mixed results. The fact that melatonin had helped a number of patients for whom all other therapies had failed—and had accomplished this feat while *improving* their quality of life—was the incentive he needed to continue working with melatonin.

► A NEW IMMUNOTHERAPY:
MELATONIN AND INTERLEUKIN-2

Over the next two years, Lissoni and his colleagues continued to conduct small clinical trials, getting slightly better results with each one. But none of their patients underwent a complete regression of their tumors. Lissoni was not surprised because he was aware that the body uses more than just melatonin to defeat cancer and other diseases—it calls on all parts of the immune system. He realized he needed to develop a therapy that came closer to duplicating the body's own multifaceted response.

In 1990 he began experimenting with just such a therapy—combining melatonin with interleukin-2. A natural component of the immune system, IL-2 is a signaling compound that stimulates the growth of the body's immune cells. For this reason, it had been under investigation as a treatment for cancer for a number of years. It was effective in treating a few kinds of cancer, primarily melanoma and renal cancer, but in the doses required to get a response, it was toxic. It was not unusual for patients to die from the treatment itself. Lissoni hoped that combining melatonin with IL-2 would allow for a much lower dose of IL-2, reducing the toxicity of the treatment without compromising its effectiveness.[20]

As he hoped, melatonin plus IL-2 proved a far superior treatment to IL-2 alone. Figure 12 compares the average immune response of ninety consecutive cancer patients who were given IL-2 plus melatonin with forty patients who were given IL-2 alone.[21] As you can see, adding melatonin to the treatment had a much greater stimulatory effect on the immune system.

The new combination therapy reduced the toxicity of IL-2 to such an extent that some of the patients were able to administer the treatment themselves at home. Each night, they would give themselves a low-dose injection of

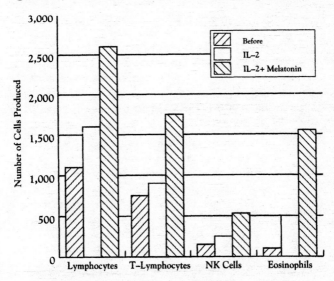

Figure 12. Melatonin Increases the Effectiveness of IL-2
When patients were given both IL-2 and melatonin, they produced more key immune cells than when given IL-2 alone. Having more of these particular immune cells is believed to increase one's chances of fighting off cancer and other diseases.

IL-2[22] and swallow a 40-milligram tablet of melatonin. This simple treatment allowed them to remain in the comfort of their own homes and saved them a great deal of money.

But how good was this home therapy? Compared with melatonin alone, melatonin plus IL-2 proved to be much more effective. More patients responded to the treatment, they experienced a greater reduction in tumor size, and for the first time, a few patients had complete regression of their tumors.

How did this therapy compare with IL-2 alone? To find out, Lissoni and his colleagues enrolled eighty patients in a randomized study.[23] IL-2 plus melatonin proved the superior treatment in every regard. For example, three patients in the IL-2 plus melatonin group underwent complete regression of their tumors, while none did in the IL-2 group. Twenty-seven percent of those given IL-2 plus melatonin had a significant reduction in tumor growth, compared with only 2 percent of the IL-2 group. In terms of survival, IL-2 plus melatonin was also clearly superior. One year after the start of the trial, 46 percent of the patients in the IL-2 plus melatonin group were still alive, compared with only 15 percent in the IL-2 group.[24]

WHAT IS A RANDOMIZED STUDY?

In a randomized study, patients are selected by lot to receive either the treatment being investigated, a placebo, and/or another kind of treatment. Assigning the patients randomly prevents the researchers from unwittingly—or wittingly—assigning healthier patients to one of the two groups. This procedure has been proven to produce more objective and accurate results.

► IL-2 PLUS MELATONIN MAY BE A SUPERIOR
   TREATMENT FOR LUNG CANCER

In a study published in 1994, Lissoni reported another significant breakthrough: He and his colleagues had demonstrated that IL-2 plus melatonin may be more effective than chemotherapy in treating an aggressive form of lung cancer called non-small-cell lung cancer. For two decades immunologists had been trying to develop a therapy to boost the immune system that was equal or superior to chemotherapy. Lissoni had just succeeded.

This particular study involved sixty patients with advanced lung cancer—a disease with a poor prognosis. Half of the patients were treated with a widely used chemotherapy regimen, cisplatin and etoposide.[25] The other half were treated with IL-2 plus melatonin. In assessing any new therapy, two main factors are considered: the quality of life of the patients after treatment, and their survival time. IL-2 plus melatonin proved superior for both factors. At the end of one year, 45 percent of those receiving the immunotherapy were still alive, compared with only 19 percent of those receiving chemotherapy. The group receiving the immunotherapy also had fewer side effects. For example, none of the patients treated with IL-2 plus melatonin experienced any vomiting, toxicity to the cardiovascular system, or blood cell abnormalities—reactions that were commonplace in the chemotherapy group.[26]

As encouraging as these results are, Lissoni believes they do not reveal the full potential of melatonin immunotherapy. His data suggests that the therapy will prove far more effective in patients in the early stages of cancer or whose immune systems have not previously been compromised by surgery, radiation, or chemotherapy. In one study, patients who had not previously been treated with chemotherapy had a 43 percent response rate to melatonin immunotherapy, while those who *had* been treated with chemotherapy had a 5 percent response rate—an eightfold difference.[27]

Lissoni awaits the day when melatonin plus IL-2 will be

approved as a first-line treatment for cancer. "Today, we work backward," he says. "First we give patients toxic therapies that cripple their immune systems. Then, if those therapies fail, we move on to therapies that *stimulate* the immune system. But that means that immunotherapists such as myself have to struggle to resuscitate an immune system that has been devastated by radiation, surgery, or chemotherapy. That does not make sense. We should start by helping the immune system do its job. If that fails, *then* we should resort to more toxic methods."

MELANOMA

Thanks in large part to the pioneering work of the Swiss and Italians, clinical oncologists in the United States are now becoming more aware of melatonin's potential. This is welcome news. Certain countries hold more sway than others in the international medical community, and the United States is one of them. Until the Swiss and Italian studies are replicated in the United States, many will discount them.

Among the Americans researching melatonin are William Robinson, M.D., and Rene Gonzalez, M.D., from the Division of Medical Oncology at the University of Colorado Health Sciences Center in Denver. Several years ago, these oncologists knew little about melatonin. Says Gonzalez, "I was taught in medical school that the pineal gland was useless. It was believed to fill up with calcium deposits as we age and thus have no known function." He remembers being skeptical of this assessment at the time. "That's not the way nature works. It doesn't go to the trouble to produce a hormone unless that hormone has a role to play."

After reading about Lissoni's cancer studies, the two men decided to launch their own clinical trial. Instead of carrying on where the Italians left off, however, they backtracked and conducted a dose-escalation trial, a study that determines the most effective dose of a given substance for a particular condition. At the time, Robinson was the director of the Melanoma Clinic at the Colorado Health Sciences Center, and he had reason to believe that melatonin might prove effective against melanoma.[28] He and Gonzalez enrolled forty-two patients with advanced melanoma for the study. On average, the patients had a life expectancy of only six months. "At this point in their treatment," says Gonzalez, "you are grasping for straws." In fact, three patients died within two weeks of joining the study.

Each day, the patients were given melatonin in tablet form, the doses ranging from a mere 5 milligrams to 700 milligrams, the largest amount ever given in a cancer study. Even at the highest dose, there were few negative side effects other than fatigue (fifteen patients) and mild nausea or diarrhea (eight patients). But the effect on tumor growth was marginal, which has been true in every study in which melatonin has been used as a solo agent. Six of the forty-two patients showed a significant reduction in tumor size. Six more had a stable condition, which means that their tumors neither grew nor shrank. Clearly, melatonin alone is not a magic bullet against cancer.

Nonetheless, a few of the patients did quite well with the treatment, two of them being women with brain metastases. Brain tumors are notoriously difficult to treat because most cancer drugs have difficulty crossing the blood-brain barrier. As you recall, melatonin does not share this limitation. One of the women who had the most dramatic response was eighty-three years old. Prior to taking part in the study, she had been treated with radiation and interferon (another experimental therapy). Neither treatment had worked, and the melanoma had invaded her brain. She was given a 50-milligram dose of melatonin in tablet form every four hours, a treatment that was without significant side effects; she suffered no nausea or hair loss and no damage to her immune system, heart, liver, or other organs. Amazingly, at the end of eight months, she had an "almost total regression of her disease."[29]

Another woman with a brain metastasis had an equally positive response. Her brain tumor was removed by surgery, after which she was given melatonin. She is alive and well four years later, a remarkable period of survival for a patient with advanced melanoma.

Robinson and Gonzalez are sufficiently encouraged by the results of their study that they plan to continue their efforts, perhaps combining melatonin with tamoxifen or using an analogue of melatonin. But the Colorado doctors have already scored a major success—alerting more oncologists to melatonin's potential. Since the publication of their study, they have gotten calls from researchers around the world who want to know more about melatonin's anticancer potential.

In the meantime, Gonzalez says he recommends melatonin to cancer patients for whom all other efforts have failed. "All they have to do," he says, "is buy five- or ten-milligram tablets at the health-food store and take them at night. The amazing thing about melatonin is that it has no toxicity. And it just might help."

To many readers, Gonzalez's recommendation will sound lukewarm: Why wait until all other treatments have failed? I must stress that before therapies based on melatonin can be approved as first-line treatments, they must be proven safe and effective in large and carefully controlled studies. So far, in the United States there has been insufficient interest and funding to conduct these studies. Lacking this assurance, few doctors, even those with personal experience with the hormone, will recommend melatonin to cancer patients except as a last resort.

CONVENTIONAL CANCER THERAPIES

In addition to its ability to enhance investigational cancer agents such as IL-2, melatonin is also proving useful in augmenting well-established cancer therapies. Exciting new data shows, for example, that melatonin may prolong the disease-free period in cancer patients who have undergone surgery.

► MELATONIN BUFFERS THE IMMUNE-SUPPRESSING EFFECTS OF SURGERY

When a patient is operated on for cancer, there is some risk that the surgery itself will help spread the tumor. The emotional stress leading up to the surgery and the physical trauma of the operation itself weaken the patient's immune system, causing a marked and persistent reduction in T cells and other immune cells.[30] During surgery, cancer cells can be dislodged and sent adrift in the patient's bloodstream. Free-floating cancer cells in a body with a weakened immune system are an invitation for metastasis. An immunotherapy that stimulated the immune system of patients before and after surgery might lower the risk of reoccurrence.

Lissoni has found that melatonin has just this effect. Working with a colleague, Fernando Brivio, he gave melatonin to thirty-five patients with advanced colorectal cancer who were scheduled to undergo surgery. (The patients were given 20 milligrams of melatonin each of the three nights leading up to their operations.) A control group was not given melatonin. Blood tests revealed that the patients receiving the hormone had a *heightened* immune response following surgery. But the real proof of the effectiveness of this treatment came two years later. Those who had been treated with melatonin had *half the rate of reoccurrence* as those who had been treated with surgery alone (20 percent versus 40 percent).[31] This is a remarkable finding. If Lissoni's results are replicated by others, giving melatonin to cancer patients in conjunction with surgery may save thousands of lives each year.

► MELATONIN COUNTERACTS THE TOXIC EFFECTS
   OF CHEMOTHERAPY

Meanwhile, Georges Maestroni has developed yet another
promising use for melatonin—to reduce the toxic effects
of chemotherapy. Most cancer drugs have a devastating
effect on the bone marrow, crippling its ability to produce
new immune cells. If the number of immune cells declines
below a critical number, chemotherapy must be delayed to
allow the body to recover. Ultimately, it matters little if
you die from cancer or from diseases brought on by a
weakened immune system. But the need to space out the
chemotherapy sessions and to limit the dosage of the drugs
compromises the effectiveness of the treatment.

One way to protect the bone marrow during chemotherapy is to give patients colony-stimulating factors,
which promote cell growth in the bone marrow. Colony-
stimulating factors are expensive to administer (costing up
to one thousand dollars per course of treatment), and they
can have negative side effects, including allergic-type reactions and bone pain.[32]

An alternative method for protecting the bone marrow
is to remove a portion of the marrow before chemotherapy
begins and then return it to the patient once the tumors
have been destroyed. (This is called an autologous transplant, meaning "from self to self.") This procedure costs
anywhere from $60,000 to $200,000, and requires that the
patient be kept in strict isolation to prevent exposure to
pathogens as the immune system recovers. This can mean
a month or more of solitude. Furthermore, the procedure
itself poses some risk: Approximately 5 percent of the patients who undergo it die from treatment-related causes.[33]

Maestroni and Conti saw a pressing need for alternative
ways to protect bone marrow during chemotherapy. In the
fall of 1994 they gave melatonin to a group of mice that
were being treated with either of two common cancer
drugs, etoposide or cyclophosphamide, both of them
highly toxic to the bone marrow. Once again, the results
were spectacular. Melatonin protected the bone marrow of

the mice *without interfering* with the cancer-fighting properties of the drugs.[34] In fact, in the parameters tested, the mice had stronger immune systems *after* chemotherapy than they did *before* being treated with the toxic chemicals! Maestroni comments, in the understated fashion common to medical researchers, "Due to the lack of undesirable side effects of melatonin, the clinical application of this finding seems straightforward."[35]

Will melatonin have the same protective effects on human cancer patients that it has had on mice? We may know within a matter of years. Augusto Pedrazzini, M.D., an oncologist practicing in Locarno, Switzerland, is conducting a pilot study in which he is giving melatonin along with chemotherapy to women with breast cancer. (The women had undergone breast surgery, but signs that the cancer had spread made chemotherapy advisable as well.)

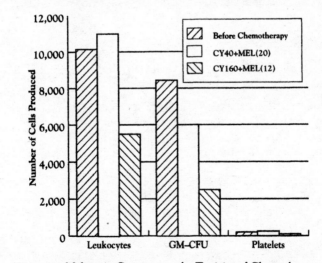

Figure 13. **Melatonin Counteracts the Toxicity of Chemotherapy**
In Maestroni's and Conti's study, giving melatonin to mice resulted in a stronger immune response after chemotherapy than before for two out of three immune indicators.

As this book goes to press, the study is still ongoing. Pedrazzini's protocol is to give the women four cycles of chemotherapy (epirubicin plus cyclophosphamide).[36] During the first and third cycles, the women are also given 20 milligrams of melatonin, which they take for seven consecutive nights. On the second and fourth cycles, they are given placebos according to the same schedule. The women do not know which pills contain melatonin and which do not.

Pedrazzini monitors the white blood cell count of the women after each cycle. He hopes that melatonin will do more than buffer the toxicity of chemotherapy—that it will actually enhance its effectiveness. Because the women have had their tumors surgically removed, however, at this time there is no way to determine if the combination therapy treatment is more or less effective than chemotherapy alone. The rate of recurrence won't be known for many years.

▶ MELATONIN AUGMENTS RADIATION THERAPY

One of the most recent findings to emerge from Italy is that melatonin may prolong the survival of patients with advanced brain cancer who are being treated with radiation. In a small pilot study, Lissoni and colleagues enrolled a group of patients with brain cancer. (The patients had malignant astrocytomas grade III-IV.) All of them were to be treated with radiation. Some of the patients were given melatonin as well. At the end of one year, three out of five patients treated with radiation plus melatonin were alive, compared with only one out of ten treated with radiation alone.[37]

Recently, I visited with Lissoni in Italy to discuss the current state of melatonin cancer therapy. A remark he made has stayed with me. "This is a very important stage in the history of medicine," he said. "We are developing a new immunotherapy for cancer that joins the forces of the immune system and the hormonal system. At the same time we are improving the quality of life of the patients. This is the future. This is the medicine of the next thousand years." From my vantage point, it appears he may be right.

CHAPTER 7

▼

PROTECTING YOUR HEART

It was two o'clock on a Friday afternoon in December 1993. I was working at the lab. I was supposed to leave in thirty minutes to pick up my wife, Nancy, at the airport, but I wasn't feeling well. I had the kind of pounding headache that you feel in your neck and temples. In my case, I knew it wasn't just a headache—it was a sign that my blood pressure was too high. Hypertension is called "the silent disease" because the condition often has no symptoms. But when your blood pressure is *really* high, believe me, you know it.

I kept hoping the headache would go away. I'd been having similar symptoms for about ten days, but they hadn't been this bad. Each time, I would tell myself, "Well, that was just an episode. Don't worry about it." But this time the headache kept getting worse and worse. I felt as if I were about to have a stroke or a heart attack. Finally I felt so strange and so ill that I walked out of my office and headed for the emergency room of the adjacent hospital, which is about a block away, through the twisting underground labyrinth of the University of Texas Health Science Center. On the way I had the vivid impression that the blood vessels in my head were about to burst.

I made it to the emergency room, found a nurse, and made a stark announcement: "I think I'm about to have a heart attack." She asked me a few questions, then took my blood pressure. It was 220 over 165, which is in the stratosphere, especially the diastolic reading. The nurse told me to lie down immediately. In a few minutes I was injected with a drug to help get my blood pressure down into a safer range. The doctor said to me, "You're lucky to be alive."

I had known I had hypertension for about ten years. From time to time, a friend who is a physician would take my blood pressure. "Russ," he would say to me, "this is bordering on treatment." Being a typical guy, I ignored him—even though both of my parents had had hypertension. In fact, my dad had a crippling stroke when he was sixty. Partly due to Nancy's influence, I began to get regular check-ups. By this time my blood pressure was high enough that it had to be treated. Unfortunately, the medications I was given were doing an inadequate job, hence the episode in 1993.

Since then, I have been taking the right combination of drugs to keep my blood pressure in the normal range. I have also begun to take melatonin. With the help of my doctor and melatonin, I may not have to suffer my father's fate.

HEART DISEASE: THE NUMBER-ONE KILLER IN THE INDUSTRIALIZED WORLD

In the United States, 59 million people are now believed to have some form of cardiovascular disease. The death rate from heart disease has declined about 25 percent in the past ten years, largely due to an increase in surgical interventions and the development of more sophisticated drugs to treat hypertension and high cholesterol. But heart disease is still our number-one killer, accounting for 42.5 percent of all deaths and a staggering $137 billion a year in heart-related medical and disability costs.[1]

Thankfully, a growing number of heart researchers have begun to focus their attention on finding ways to *prevent* heart disease, not just treat it. Antioxidant therapy is showing considerable promise. A number of studies have shown that taking antioxidant vitamins—or better yet, eating foods rich in antioxidants—decreases blood pressure, lowers cholesterol, and reduces the incidence of heart disease.[2] There is also evidence that some foods lower cholesterol, especially soy and oat products.

But to my mind, some of the most exciting work is being done by researchers studying the body's own mechanisms for maintaining a healthy heart. Having a functioning heart is essential for survival, and any function that is necessary for life is well provided for in the overall design of the human body—at least in the young. Researchers believe that if they can gain more insight into those natural mechanisms, they might be able to help sustain them into old age.

THE HEART AT NIGHT

With this goal in mind, a few researchers have begun to study how the heart functions at night. The cardiovascular system, it has been known for some time, has a distinct daily cycle. During the nighttime, your heart beats more slowly, your blood pressure drops, and the amount of cholesterol in your bloodstream declines. On a cellular level, an enzyme called the calcium pump becomes more active, purging the cells of excess calcium.[3]

As day breaks, your heart picks up its pace, your blood pressure rises, and the level of calcium builds up in your cells. These changes help you gear up for the challenges of the day, but at the same time they also increase your risk of heart attack and stroke, especially as you age. Statistics show you are most vulnerable to a cardiac emergency between six A.M. and twelve noon, with the greatest risk occurring around nine A.M.[4] Among themselves, some heart specialists refer to these morning hours as the "heart attack zone."

Why is your heart better behaved at night? At first you might think that it's just because you are lying down and sleeping, lowering your level of physical activity. This is not the full explanation. In a number of studies, volunteers have been kept awake under constant lighting conditions for twenty-four hours at a stretch. Typically, they are asked to sit in a chair or recline on a bed and engage in a quiet activity such as reading, watching TV, or playing cards. They are offered a meal every four hours around the clock. The researchers staffing the study are careful to interact with the patients to the same degree night and day and to make sure that the patients stay awake and maintain the same level of physical activity. Yet even under these carefully controlled conditions, the patients have lower blood pressure, pulse rate, and cholesterol levels at night. What drives this circadian rhythm?

An obvious candidate is melatonin. As we have seen, your body produces more melatonin at night. Interestingly, your blood pressure and pulse rate reach the low point of the twenty-four-hour cycle at the same time your melatonin levels peak, around two or three in the morning. Furthermore, the "heart attack zone" occurs at about the time your melatonin levels reach their daytime low. Is this coincidence, or is it cause and effect?

Melatonin appears in fact to have a *direct* protective effect on the heart and the circulatory system in general. What's more, there is growing evidence that declining levels of melatonin—both the abrupt fall that occurs in the morning and the gradual overall decline that accompanies aging—are hazardous to the heart. In the pages that follow, I'll present striking new evidence showing that melatonin contributes to nearly every aspect of heart health.

MELATONIN REDUCES CHOLESTEROL

High cholesterol is a known risk factor for atherosclerosis, the narrowing, thickening, and loss of elasticity of the arteries. One of the primary causes of atherosclerosis is a buildup of LDL cholesterol, the "bad" cholesterol that ferries fatty acids from your liver to your arteries. If enough cholesterol accumulates in a vital artery, the flow of blood to the heart or brain becomes blocked. Fifty-two percent of all Americans have cholesterol levels over 200, increasing their risk of heart attack and stroke.[5] One way to lower your cholesterol is to reduce your intake of fatty foods such as eggs, butter, cheese, and meat. Exercise helps as well. But if your level is very high (over 250), your doctor is likely to recommend cholesterol-lowering medications as well. In the future, melatonin may be one of the substances he or she prescribes.

Japanese researchers have learned a great deal about melatonin's effects on cholesterol. In three studies conducted in the 1980s, they found that the hormone reduced the cholesterol levels of rats that had high cholesterol for one of three reasons—heredity,[6] a fatty diet,[7] or drug manipulation.[8] In the experiment involving hereditary high cholesterol, the investigators found that melatonin also "greatly reduced the fatty development in the liver."[9]

A group of Italian researchers have further demonstrated the link between melatonin and cholesterol. In one experiment, the investigators removed the pineal glands of four-month-old mice, eliminating their nightly production of melatonin. When the rodents reached adulthood, their cholesterol levels were 30 percent higher than normal. In another study, melatonin was given to aging mice and the hormone prevented the age-related increase in cholesterol.[10]

In 1994 a group of German scientists became curious about the effect of melatonin on human cholesterol production. They were prompted by a finding from one of their earlier studies that people with high levels of LDL cholesterol had low levels of melatonin.[11] To see if melatonin has a direct effect on cholesterol production, they incubated human white blood cells in various concentrations of the hormone. Melatonin blocked the formation of cholesterol by as much as 38 percent. It also caused a 42 percent reduction in LDL accumulation.[12]

New data shows that people who take melatonin have a significant drop in cholesterol. One of the findings to emerge from the B-Oval contraceptive study (see Chapter 6) is that the fourteen hundred women taking the melatonin-based pill have significantly lower cholesterol levels than they did before joining the study. According to the originator of the pill, Michael Cohen, M.D., "There is a 10-20 percent reduction in cholesterol across the board in the women who use the B-Oval pill."[13] James W. Anderson, M.D., chief of the endocrine-metabolic section at the Veterans Affairs Medical Center in Lexington, Kentucky, believes this reduction in cholesterol could cause a significant reduction in their risk of heart disease. He says,

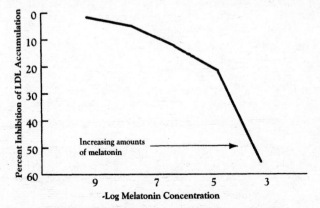

Figure 14. Melatonin Decreases LDL Cholesterol

"Even a 10 to 15 percent reduction in blood cholesterol results in a 20 to 30 percent reduction in the risk of coronary artery disease."[14]

This is good news for people with high cholesterol. The drugs currently being used to lower cholesterol can have numerous side effects, including liver damage, muscle inflammation, allergic reaction, and headache.[15] Melatonin—nature's own remedy—could prove to be a safer (and less expensive) course of action.

ADDING ANTIOXIDANT PROTECTION

Lowering your cholesterol levels is just one part of a comprehensive program to lower your risk of atherosclerosis. You may also need to boost your antioxidant protection. A relatively new insight is that a high level of LDL cholesterol in and of itself may not lead to clogged arteries. It could be that before LDL can adhere to the flattened cells (called endothelial cells) that line your arteries, it has to be damaged by free radicals.

LDL cholesterol is packaged in fatty compartments called lipoproteins, which are prime targets for free-radical damage. When the lipoproteins become damaged, immune cells swarm to envelop them and cart them away. The result is a population of sticky globs of cholesterol that can cling to the linings of your arteries, forming swollen yellow mounds known as plaque. If other damaged lipoproteins add their cargo of cholesterol to the plaque, it can choke off the artery. (The surgical procedure called balloon angioplasty is designed to remove the plaque with an inflatable tool.)

Antioxidants reduce the oxidation of LDL cholesterol and prevent it from adhering to artery walls. In a recent study, a group of monkeys was fed a high-fat diet, and another group the same diet enriched with a potent antioxidant (probucol). The monkeys with the added antioxidant protection had much healthier arteries.[16]

Antioxidants appear to have the same beneficial effect on monkeys' human cousins. A study published in *The Journal of the American Medical Association* in 1995 showed that men who took at least 100 IU of vitamin E every day had less damage to their arteries than those who consumed smaller amounts of the antioxidant vitamin.[17] Given that melatonin may be at least twice as effective as vitamin E at preventing free radical damage, it is likely to provide the same or even greater benefit.[18]

CORONARY HEART DISEASE

Additional evidence linking melatonin with a healthy heart comes from a study published in *Lancet* in 1995. In this study, researchers from Vienna compared the nighttime melatonin levels of a group of ten healthy volunteers with a group of fifteen patients with coronary heart disease. (Coronary heart disease occurs when there is an insufficient flow of blood to the heart muscle; the most common cause of this disease is atherosclerosis.) The two groups were matched for sex and age, eliminating two possible confounding factors. The results showed that the people with healthy hearts were producing *five times* as much melatonin as those with diseased hearts.[19]

The paper concluded: "Because melatonin concentration can be increased by oral administration of melatonin, it would be easy to treat patients with coronary heart disease with melatonin to study effects on the development of atherosclerosis and coronary heart disease."[20] It is my fervent hope that such a study will soon be under way.

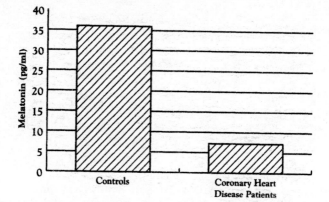

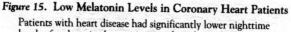

Figure 15. **Low Melatonin Levels in Coronary Heart Patients**
Patients with heart disease had significantly lower nighttime
levels of melatonin than patients without heart disease.

HYPERTENSION

When it comes to high blood pressure, I have a lot of
company. Approximately 50 million people in the United
States have hypertension, a known risk factor for heart
disease and stroke. (High blood pressure is defined as having systolic blood pressure over 140 and/or diastolic blood
pressure over 90.) Despite the great number of people afflicted with this condition, its underlying causes are not
well understood. In fact, 90 percent of all cases are attributed to unknown causes.[21]

Like the risk for high cholesterol, the risk for hypertension increases with age. Is it possible that the age-related
decline in melatonin production is one "unknown cause"
of hypertension? The first data supporting this contention
came from early observations of pinealectomized animals.
As far back as the 1960s, it was known that animals deprived of their pineal glands have higher blood pressure.
(This condition is referred to as pinealectomy-induced hypertension.)

In 1975 a researcher discovered that if he gave melatonin to pinealectomized animals, their blood pressure went down—in some instances *to below normal levels*. When he stopped giving them melatonin, their blood pressure shot back up, indicating a cause-and-effect relationship between blood pressure and melatonin.[22]

Further evidence of a melatonin-blood pressure connection comes from studies involving the "spontaneously hypertensive rat," a peculiar strain of laboratory rat that develops high blood pressure at the tender age of three months. These rats have an unusual pattern of melatonin production. They produce relatively high amounts of the hormone for the first three months of life; then for some unknown reason, their levels plunge to below normal, at which time the rats become hypertensive. The adults have melatonin levels 50 percent lower than other rat strains.[23]

HYPERTENSION AND MELATONIN IN HUMANS

These findings raise an obvious question: Do people with high blood pressure have low melatonin levels? It is not easy to find the answer because most people with hypertension are over 40 years old and are likely to have declining levels of melatonin simply because of their age. Several studies have shown, however, that for adults matched for age, those with hypertension have lower melatonin levels than those with normal blood pressure.[24] Also, in a 1988 Scandinavian study, people with severe hypertension had half the nighttime melatonin levels of people with moderate hypertension.[25]

Such findings are regarded as indirect evidence because they do not *prove* that melatonin has a direct effect on blood pressure; they merely show a correlation. But there is preliminary evidence that melatonin does help regulate blood pressure in humans. In 1980 a researcher named Nicholas Birau, M.D., conducted a double-blind study in which he administered melatonin to twenty patients with high blood pressure. Every afternoon for one week, Birau gave the patients either of two different nose drop preparations—one that contained melatonin, and one that did not.[26] The next week, each patient received the alternate treatment. (This is called a crossover study because after a period of time, each patient "crosses over" to the other treatment.) At no time did either Birau or the patients know which preparation was being administered.

When the study was over, Birau reported that when the volunteers were taking the nose drops that did not contain melatonin, their blood pressure remained abnormally high. But when they were taking the melatonin nose drops, their blood pressure declined to within the normal range.[27]

Further evidence of melatonin's blood-pressure-lowering ability comes from the B-Oval trial. Michael Cohen reports that the women taking the pill have had a reduction in blood pressure: "During the medication period, there was a slight yet highly significant decrease in diastolic and systolic blood pressure from 116 over 76.3 to 107.4 over 71.2; this effect was reversed after cessation of the medication."[28]

Meanwhile, anecdotal evidence of melatonin's effect on blood pressure is coming from the largest study of all—the unstructured study involving all the hundreds of thousands of people who are now taking melatonin on their own. A colleague of mine at UTHSC, a forty-eight-year-old woman, has been taking melatonin for about a year and a half. Two years ago her blood pressure was 140 over 104—making her borderline hypertensive. Recently, she had her blood pressure taken, for the first time since being on melatonin. Her reading was 128 over 68, a significant drop. It is even more impressive considering that for much of the time she had been taking a very low-dose melatonin tablet, 0.3 milligrams (not the 3-milligram tablets commonly sold in health-food stores). "The nurse asked me if I was on antihypertensive medicine," she told me. "I told her I wasn't. She said she wanted to come back and retest me in ten minutes. The second time she took my blood

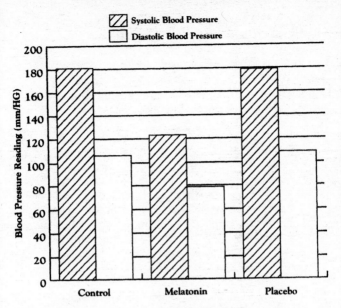

Figure 16. Melatonin May Reduce High Blood Pressure
Patients with high blood pressure who were given melatonin
nose drops had a significant drop in blood pressure within
one week. When the same patients were given placebo nose
drops, their blood pressure did not change.

pressure, it was 124 over 65. She said to me, 'Whatever
you're doing, keep on doing it.'"

How does melatonin affect blood pressure? There are
three possible mechanisms. One is that the hormone acts
directly on the hypothalamus, an area deep in the brain
that regulates blood pressure and is known to be rich with
melatonin receptors. Another and more recent explanation is that melatonin lowers blood pressure through its
antioxidant effects. Several studies have shown that antioxidants lower blood pressure.[29] Interestingly, antioxidants seem to have a marked effect only in people with
hypertension, and the same may be true for melatonin.
When Birau gave the melatonin nose drops to people

without hypertension, their blood pressure remained essentially unchanged. Finally, melatonin may link with receptors on arterial walls, causing the arteries to expand. This third possible mechanism was presented by L. Bruce Weekley, Ph.D., in *The Journal of Pineal Research* in 1991. In a study of rats, Weekley found that melatonin relaxes the smooth muscle lining the aorta.[30]

HOW DO ANTIOXIDANTS LOWER BLOOD PRESSURE?

The blood vessels are lined with a layer of endothelial cells that secrete *relaxing factors*, which cause the vessels to expand, thus lowering blood pressure. One such relaxing factor is nitric oxide. Nitric oxide is rapidly inactivated by a free radical called the superoxide radical. Increasing your antioxidant protection reduces the number of superoxide radicals, which spares nitric oxide and allows the blood vessels to expand. The net result is lower blood pressure.

Twenty-five million Americans are now taking high blood pressure medications. The medications most commonly used—diuretics, beta-blockers, calcium antagonists, and ACE inhibitors—can cause a number of negative side effects, including high blood sugar, depression, elevated LDL cholesterol, increased risk of cardiac arrhythmia, impotence, potassium deficiency, and asthma.[31]

Calcium channel blockers and ACE inhibitors are considerably more expensive than older hypertensive medications such as diuretics and beta-blockers, which means they can also have a negative effect on your pocketbook. A greater reliance on these drugs has increased the nation's health care bill by an estimated $10 billion a year.[32] If melatonin or a closely related substance is proven to be a safe, effective, low-cost treatment for hypertension, the nation might save billions of health care dollars, tens of thousands of lives and an untold amount of human suffering.

If you are currently taking anti-hypertensive medication, however, you should continue doing so. The medication may be preventing a heart attack or stroke. There is no evidence at this time that melatonin can replace traditional heart medications. The data is merely suggestive.

BLOOD CLOTS

Platelets are small cell fragments that are formed in the bone marrow and that circulate throughout the bloodstream to help guard against the loss of blood. When a blood vessel is injured, platelets clump together to help seal the breach. A careful balance must be maintained, however. If your platelets become too sticky, they may clump together unnecessarily and block a vital artery; if they become too slick, they will no longer function as a Band-Aid, and you might run the risk of uncontrolled bleeding. Your body has worked out a clever compromise between these alternatives. During the daytime, when your risk of physical injury is highest, your platelets are more likely to clump together. When you are safely tucked away in bed, your platelets are less sticky, lowering your risk of heart attack and stroke without putting you at undue risk.

There is reason to believe that this compromise is mediated by your nocturnal rise in melatonin. When human blood platelets are incubated in a melatonin solution, the hormone reduces their tendency to clump by as much as 85 percent.[33] Here is yet another avenue of research which could lead to better and safer heart medications.

HEART ATTACK

One of the new insights to come from the burgeoning field of free-radical research is that free radicals add to the havoc caused by acute heart disease. During a heart attack or stroke, portions of the heart or brain are deprived of the life-giving flow of blood, damaging the tissues through oxygen starvation. When the blood seeps back into the damaged area, a great number of free radicals are created, which can cause further damage.[34] (This is the reperfusion injury that occurs during strokes, as we saw in Chapter 3.)

How do we know that free radicals play a role in heart attacks? Scientists discovered that free radicals play a role in reperfusion injury by measuring the amount of pentane gas exhaled by recent heart attack victims. Pentane is a hydrocarbon gas that is a by-product of free-radical damage to the cell membranes. Eventually, pentane collects in the lungs and is exhaled. The more pentane exhaled, the more free-radical damage is taking place somewhere in the body. A recent study showed that people who have suffered a heart attack within the past twelve hours exhale almost three times as much pentane as people hospitalized for other reasons.[35]

To a lesser degree, the same damaging process takes place during most heart operations, including transplant surgery, bypass surgery, and even balloon angioplasty. Anytime that blood is blocked from your heart and then flows back in, free radicals are produced, which cause some amount of tissue damage. To minimize this damage, heart specialists have begun to give antioxidants to their patients before surgery, and a growing number of hospitals are adding antioxidants to the blood supply before transfusing it into a heart patient. Will there soon come a day when melatonin is added to the blood supply as well?

HEARTBEAT IRREGULARITIES

Each year more than 3.5 million Americans experience an episode of heartbeat irregularity, or arrhythmia. If the heart's rhythm becomes so disordered that the heart loses its ability to pump blood, death can come in a matter of minutes. Heart arrhythmia causes the death of more than forty thousand Americans each year.

Heart arrhythmia, like most heart problems, occurs less frequently at night than during the day. Anytime a bodily function has a distinct circadian rhythm, there is reason to think that melatonin, the body's timekeeper, might be involved. Researchers at the Cardiovascular Research Laboratories at Harvard University have found such a connection for heart arrhythmia. Applying a mild electrical current to the hearts of laboratory animals can trigger arrhythmia; the amount of current it takes to do so is a measure of the heart's electrical stability. The higher the electrical stability of the heart, the less likely the current will cause arrhythmia.

In the Harvard study, researchers gave injections of melatonin to a group of dogs, then measured the amount of current required to destabilize their hearts. The melatonin-treated dogs required 28 percent more current than dogs not given the heart-calming hormone.[36] These findings had "profound clinical implications," the researchers concluded.

They made another interesting observation: There is a high incidence of arrhythmias in patients admitted to intensive care units (ICUs), even when the patients do not have preexisting heart problems. Knowing that bright light can inhibit the body's production of melatonin (a topic I will explore in Chapter 13), the researchers speculated that the continuous lighting in ICUs might lower patients' melatonin levels, thereby reducing the electrical stability of their hearts and making them more vulnerable to arrhythmia.

If this is so, a simple way to lower the risk is to provide

patients with sleep masks to shield their eyes during the night, thus preserving their life-giving supply of melatonin.

WILL TAKING MELATONIN LOWER *YOUR* RISK OF HEART DISEASE?

Given the preliminary evidence that melatonin reduces cholesterol, inhibits the oxidation of LDL cholesterol, helps maintain normal blood pressure, reduces the tendency of blood platelets to clump, and stabilizes the electrical activity of the heart, there is reason to believe that maintaining a youthful supply of melatonin could lower the risk of heart disease.

If you have heart problems—or want to *prevent* heart problems—should you take melatonin? A definitive answer can come only from carefully controlled studies. The evidence presented in this chapter is preliminary and inconclusive. But it is suggestive enough that researchers must now go on to answer these questions. The fact that a naturally produced, nontoxic hormone may help lower the risk of heart disease—helping to save lives, preserve the quality of life for hundreds of thousands of people, and lower our astronomical health care costs—is one of the most promising findings to come out of any field of medical research in recent decades.

CHAPTER 8

▼

UNLOCKING THE SLEEP GATE

Jean L., 69, credits melatonin with rescuing her from a thirteen-year struggle with insomnia. She developed sleeping problems after having a hysterectomy at the age of 55. Following the operation she had great difficulty sleeping, getting only three to four hours of sleep a night. She became desperate for sleep: "I am in the retail clothing business, and I was interacting with eight hundred customers a week. I really had to be on the ball. I got so I couldn't remember names, even people I knew really well. I couldn't think of what to say from one minute to the next. Everyone could see that something was really wrong with me."

Jean finally went to her doctor, who gave her a prescription for a sleeping medication called triazolam (Halcion). It helped her sleep from the very start. "It was a goody," she says. "It was very fast acting, and it helped me sleep through the night." She took Halcion for three years. Then one day without warning, her doctor refused to write her another prescription. "He told me they were finding all these bad things with Halcion," she says, "so he didn't want me to take it anymore."

Immediately, Jean's insomnia returned, only now it was worse than before. She had an added problem as well—she felt deeply depressed. "No one had told me that I wouldn't be able to sleep once I went off the drug," she says, "or that I would feel so depressed." She turned to over-the-counter sleeping pills for relief. "I was on those antihistamines for two years," she says. "Then my heart started pounding at night, so I figured they must be bad for you, too. I went back to my doctor, and that's when he told me about melatonin."

Jean tried melatonin and found that it worked remarkably well. "It didn't knock me out like Halcion, but it gave me an even better sleep. I take the kind that you dissolve under your tongue. Sometimes I'm asleep before it's all the way dissolved. When I wake up, I don't feel groggy or druggy. With melatonin, you don't know that you've taken anything."

Jean has noticed a lot of changes since taking melatonin. "When you sleep better, everything works better. My memory has improved. I have more energy. And my sex life is great, even after forty-two years of marriage."

Jean is one of a growing number of people worldwide who are taking melatonin to get a better night's sleep. The general public first learned that melatonin is a remedy for insomnia in the fall of 1993. Highly publicized results of a sleep study conducted at the Massachusetts Institute of Technology (MIT) revealed that a mere trace of melatonin—0.1 milligrams—enhanced sleep in healthy young volunteers.[1]

Researchers, however, have known about melatonin's sleep-enhancing effects for decades. The first person to get a hint of them was Aaron Lerner, the Yale dermatologist who discovered melatonin. In 1960, when he injected the hormone into a human subject for the first time, he observed that the volunteer experienced a mild sedation. Before long, other researchers were experimenting with this new and mysterious substance. Their one consistent finding was that it made subjects feel relaxed or sleepy. At first, they thought melatonin's sedative property was a side effect, akin to the drowsiness caused by antihistamines. Now it is believed that inducing sleep is one of the hormone's primary roles.[2]

WHO HAS SLEEP PROBLEMS?

The number of people who might benefit from taking melatonin as a sleep aid is enormous. In the United States approximately one out of every four adults and two out of every four senior citizens have trouble falling asleep or staying asleep. Women as a group have more difficulty sleeping than men, partly because of the effects of menstruation, pregnancy, nursing, child care, and menopause.

The financial toll exacted by insomnia is overwhelming. The National Commission on Sleep Disorders estimates that we spend at least $16 billion a year on problems directly associated with sleep disorders. This figure does not include the indirect costs of accidents caused by sleep-deprived people. The figure is likely to rise even further in the years to come as baby boomers enter their golden years. By the year 2010, an estimated 79 million Americans will be at risk for chronic sleep difficulties.[3]

Judging from recent studies, a high percentage of the old and restless can benefit from taking melatonin. Researchers at the Oregon Health Sciences University (OHSU) are in the midst of a five-year, $5 million study of the effects of melatonin on sleep. According to Cliff Singer, M.D., one of the principal researchers, their findings have been very positive: "We have preliminary data showing that melatonin is just as effective as a common prescription sleep aid but, unlike that drug, does *not* interfere with the quality of sleep. When you add to this the fact that melatonin is a potent antioxidant and strengthens the immune system, the implications are boundless."

An Israeli colleague agrees with Singer's assessment. Peretz Lavie, M.D., dean of medicine at the Israel Institute of Technology in Haifa, told a reporter for *The New York Times* that melatonin "works better than I dreamed possible." In one of the studies in which Lavie was involved, insomniacs were given 2 milligrams of melatonin two hours before bedtime. After one week of therapy, according to Lavie, "they slept much, much better."

THE PROS AND CONS OF CURRENT SLEEP MEDICATIONS

Melatonin's sleep-enhancing properties are all the more impressive when compared with those of current sleep aids. The most commonly used remedy for insomnia is found not in the medicine cabinet but in the liquor cabinet. An estimated 20 percent of insomniacs rely on alcohol to relax their muscles, ease their anxiety, and help them fall asleep. But alcohol is not a very good sleep aid for a number of reasons, chief among them the fact that it fractures sleep. A nightcap may help you fall asleep more quickly, but several hours later the alcohol will have a rebound effect, making you restless and maybe even agitated in the second half of the night. In the end, you sleep worse than if you had not taken the drink.

Another large segment of the sleep-deprived population turns to over-the-counter medications. The active ingredient in most of these preparations is either diphenhydramine or doxylamine, antihistamines that cause drowsiness as a side effect. These medications may help with mild or occasional sleeplessness, but they're not recommended for chronic use, especially for those with glaucoma, peptic ulcer, bronchial asthma, seizures, or prostate enlargement. They may also cause a number of side effects, including dry mouth, increased heart rate, and next-day drowsiness. (Doxylamine, for example, has a half-life of nine hours. This means that if you take one of the tablets at eleven P.M., you will still have significant amounts in your bloodstream at eight A.M.[4]) Furthermore, many people find that the antihistamine-based preparations are not potent enough to resolve serious sleep difficulties or nighttime anxiety.

When insomniacs turn to their doctors for help, more often than not they are given a prescription for a benzodiazepine (pronounced "ben-zoe-die-AZ-a-peen"), a family of drugs that includes Dalmane, Doral, Halcion, ProSom, Restoril, Valium, and Xanax. Twenty million prescriptions are written in the United States for these drugs each year.[5] To a person desperate for sleep, they can seem a godsend. They are less toxic than the barbiturates people commonly took years ago, and they are less likely to cause dependency. They can be very effective in helping you fall asleep more quickly, reducing the number of times you awaken, and increasing your total sleep time. They are especially beneficial for anxiety-related insomnia.

But benzodiazepines have a number of limitations. The longer-acting ones, such as Dalmane, can cause next-day drowsiness. Halcion, a very short-acting benzodiazepine, has been associated with a number of negative side effects, including depression and anxiety. Some researchers question whether the product should remain on the market at all.[6] In addition, mixing some of these drugs with alcohol can have toxic effects.[7]

There's another problem with benzodiazepines: Many can cause a specific kind of memory loss called anterograde amnesia. You might not retain any memories of what happened while you were under the influence of these drugs. For example, many people take benzodiazepines to help them sleep during a long plane flight. There are numerous reports of people who have awakened the next morning in a strange hotel room, with no memory of getting off the plane or finding their way to the hotel. (This phenomenon is most likely to occur when other factors are involved, such as sleep deprivation, alcohol, and/or jet lag.)[8]

One way researchers determine if a sleep medication

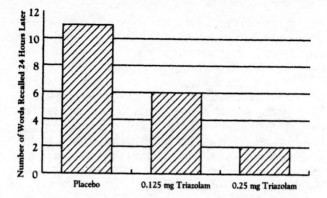

Figure 17. **A Common Sleep Medication Impairs Memory**
When volunteers were given the sleep medication triazolam
(Halcion), they recalled fewer words from a random list read to
them a day earlier. The higher the dose of the medication, the
worse their memory.

interferes with memory is to administer the drug to volunteers, wait two hours, then read them a list of unrelated
words. The next day, the volunteers are asked to recall as
many of those words as they can. The graph in Figure 17
shows the average number of words recalled by twenty-six
volunteers after taking either a placebo or Halcion in one
of two different doses.[9] This diminution of memory is one
of the reasons that the military has banned the use of most
benzodiazepines. They cannot risk having key personnel
with impaired memory.

THE STAGES OF SLEEP

A more fundamental problem with benzodiazepines is that
they can interfere with normal sleep. Researchers have
found that the mysterious process of sleep can be divided
into five separate stages. Stage I sleep is the shallow sleep
you experience upon falling asleep. You may porpoise in
and out of stage I sleep—sometimes awake, sometimes half

asleep—until you finally surrender. Rather quickly you descend to stage II sleep, which some researchers regard as the first true sleep. You rest in stage II, then sink to the lower levels, III and IV. By now, about 45 minutes have passed.

Stages III and IV are also referred to as slow wave sleep or delta sleep because they are characterized by slow brain waves called delta waves. The immune system appears to be most active during slow wave sleep.[10] Many people are deficient in slow wave sleep, including most older people, pain sufferers, people who take certain sleeping pills, and those with chronic fatigue syndrome or fibromyalgia. A common problem among these people is that they feel sleepy or fatigued throughout the day and are more susceptible to viral and bacterial infections.

You dwell in these subterranean depths for a period of time, then you climb back up the stages until you crest at Stage I again and then begin your first cycle of dreaming, or REM sleep. (REM stands for "rapid eye movement," a term that researchers coined when they noted that when people dream, their eyes dart to and fro as if they were watching a private screening of a movie.) After a period of

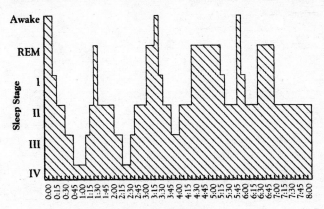

Figure 18. The Stages of Sleep

dreaming, you sink back down the stages. You repeat this elevator ride several times during the night, but you spend more time in deep sleep in the first half of the night than you do in the second. This may be nature's way of insuring that you get enough deep sleep, which appears to be essential for your health and well-being.

When graphed on a chart such as the one in Figure 18, the stages of sleep resemble a city landscape, which may be why the overall pattern of sleep is referred to as "sleep architecture."

When you take a nap during the daytime, your sleep is similar to your sleep at night. Since naps are shorter, however, you don't have time to cycle through all the stages. A twenty-minute nap, for example, may take you no farther than stage I or II sleep. When you wake up, you are likely to feel refreshed and alert. But if you take a longer nap— long enough to sink into slow wave sleep but not long enough to make your way back up—you may wake up feeling groggy and disoriented, a phenomenon known as sleep inertia. It will be some time before your brain cycles back to the shorter wavelengths typical of an awake and alert frame of mind.[11] You may wish you had not taken that nap.

MOST SLEEP REMEDIES DISRUPT THE STAGES OF SLEEP

An ideal sleep aid is one that preserves normal sleep architecture. Few match this description. Alcohol and most benzodiazepines, for example, reduce the amount of time you spend dreaming. A deficiency of REM sleep can cause memory problems and varying degrees of physical and psychic disturbance. In fact, animals that are kept from dreaming several weeks in a row may die prematurely.

Benzodiazepines can also shortchange stages III and IV sleep. Taking one of these drugs for months at a time can abolish the deeper levels of sleep altogether.[12] For this and other reasons, benzodiazepines are not recommended for long-term use. They help you get to sleep and stay asleep, but they may result in a pseudosleep that restores neither body nor soul.

Drug manufacturers themselves warn against taking these products for long periods of time, yet some people (like Jean) take them for months or even years. Doctors who prescribe several months' worth of sleeping pills at a time promote this misuse—and many do. More than a third of the prescriptions for benzodiazepines written for people over 65 provide a six-month supply or more.[13] A friend of mine who is a sleep researcher believes that the abuse of benzodiazepines is rampant. At a recent conference on sleep, he told me, a doctor stood up and said to the assembled group, "Who are we kidding? We know that these drugs are supposed to be given for only two or three weeks, but I'm telling you every person here prescribes benzodiazepines for some patients for years. We need something better."

When people take sleep medications for months at a time, they are likely to become resistant to them and require higher doses to relieve their insomnia. Eventually they may become dependent on the drugs. If they try to withdraw, they are likely to experience rebound anxiety, a reaction typified by anxiety, fatigue, insomnia, and irritability. The temptation to go back on the pills can be strong.

MELATONIN—NO KNOWN ADVERSE SIDE-EFFECTS

Melatonin has none of the negative side effects associated with traditional sleep medications. To begin with, it does not significantly disrupt the sleep architecture. In 1974 a group of researchers concluded: "Melatonin-induced sleep, behaviorally as well as by its polygraphic pattern, strikingly resembles natural sleep."[14] Subsequent studies have supported this finding.

Nor does nature's sleeping pill interfere with a person's memory or performance the next day. In an afternoon sleep study conducted at Bowling Green State University in Ohio, a group of young men were assigned randomly to receive either a 1-, 10-, or 40-milligram dose of melatonin.[15] The men took their pills and then two hours later were encouraged to take a nap. Four hours later, all of the men who had taken the 40-milligram dose were still sound asleep and had to be awakened. Shortly after awakening, the men were given tests of their performance, memory, and fatigue. According to one of the investigators, Rod Hughes, Ph.D., "Test results suggested that melatonin had no carry-over fatigue and no negative effects on memory or performance. This is quite different from what you see with most benzodiazepines."[16]

Nor does melatonin appear to have negative side effects in the elderly. This finding is important because older people as a group tend to be more sensitive to the negative effects of all medications, including sleep medications. In a study conducted in 1994 at OHSU a group of healthy elderly people (average age 84.5 years) were given 50 milligrams of melatonin, a very high dose. But not even this amount interfered with their memory, concentration, or motor control.[17]

Another reason that melatonin is such a superlative sleep aid is that it does not lose its effectiveness over time. Benzodiazepines can become less effective after only two or three nights of use. By contrast, melatonin may become a *more* effective sleep aid with chronic use. In an Israeli study, researchers gave 2-milligram doses of melatonin to elderly volunteers for two months. At the end of the treatment period, the volunteers fell asleep even more quickly than they did after one week of treatment.[18]

This finding is of great import for the elderly. Most older people with insomnia have *chronic*, not temporary sleep problems, yet the existing prescription medications are not recommended for chronic use. Until now, the elderly have had to choose between restless nights and abusing their medications.

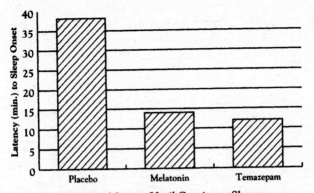

Figure 19. Minutes Until Consistent Sleep
In this pilot study, volunteers who took melatonin fell asleep
almost as quickly as those given a potent sleep medication.

IS MELATONIN AN *EFFECTIVE* SLEEP AID?

Melatonin may be a safe and natural sleep aid, but is it
effective? Once again, the answer appears to be yes. High
doses of melatonin can have dramatic sleep-inducing effects. In a study conducted at Brooks Air Force Base in
San Antonio, volunteers arrived at a sleep lab early in the
morning after a full night's rest. At nine o'clock, each
volunteer was given a pill containing one of three preparations—a placebo or 10 or 100 milligrams of melatonin.
The volunteers were then free to visit, read, or play video
games. Every two hours, they were subjected to a battery
of tests. Around noon, one of the volunteers who had
received the 100-milligram dose began playing a video
football game. He was an ace player and was winning all
his games. During one close game he managed to maneu-
ver his running back close to the goal line. Unfortunately,
he fell asleep just as his player reached the five-yard line.
His opponent gleefully seized the opportunity to tackle
the player, preventing a game-winning touchdown.[19]

Doses as small as 10 milligrams can also have profound
sleep-enhancing effects. A sleep researcher tells about a

physician who worked the night shift one Friday night. The physician went home Saturday morning, took 10 milligrams of melatonin, and went to bed. He slept all day, woke up, ate dinner, and went back to bed, soaking up a total of nineteen hours of sleep.[20]

Amazingly, even fractions of a milligram of melatonin can enhance sleep. Richard Wurtman, M.D., a longtime colleague of mine from MIT, demonstrated this fact in a series of studies that spanned ten years. In the early years of melatonin sleep research, it was thought that melatonin induced sleep only in very high doses. So in one of Wurtman's first studies, he administered 240 milligrams of the hormone, an extremely high dose by today's terms. Not surprisingly, the volunteers felt sleepy and fatigued.[21] Nine years later, his group conducted a similar experiment using much smaller doses—80, 40, 20, and 10 milligrams. They found that all of these doses, even the 10-milligram dose, had a potent soporific effect as well.

These results made them curious about just how small a dose would make people sleepy. In a study published in 1995, they gave volunteers either 1-milligram or 0.3-milligram doses of melatonin. Even these minute quantities decreased the amount of time it took volunteers to fall asleep, the smaller dose being just as effective as the larger one.[22]

OVERCOMING "SPACE SHUTTLE LAG"

Melatonin sleep research has come to the attention of a number of government agencies, including the National Aeronautics and Space Administration (NASA). Recently, I was invited to give a lecture on melatonin at the NASA/Johnson Space Center in Houston. The researchers wanted to know all they could about the versatile hormone because they thought it might help astronauts deal with some of the problems they encounter in space, especially "Space Shuttle lag" and insomnia.

Most astronauts have sleep problems, and for very good reason, I learned. In the days leading up to the launch, they are very excited about the upcoming mission and, understandably, a little nervous as well. The closer they get to launch time, records show, the less they sleep. Once in space additional concerns keep them awake, like the fact that they are under constant pressure to perform at peak levels. Given the enormous cost of a space mission, an astronaut's time is calculated to be worth approximately $20,000 an hour,[23] a level of responsibility that might keep anyone awake.

But even without pressure of this kind, astronauts would find it difficult to sleep. The Space Shuttle circles the globe every ninety minutes, exposing them to a dizzying succession of forty-five-minute days and forty-five-minute nights. Maintaining a normal sleep schedule under these conditions is no small feat. Then there's the novelty of sleeping in zero gravity. Even a simple hand movement, astronauts complain, can make them knock against the overhead bunk, waking up a crewmate.

For these reasons and more, most astronauts have difficulty getting a full night's sleep, increasing their risk of making a costly error or, worse yet, compromising the mission.[24] The present policy is to give astronauts benzodiazepines to help them sleep, but NASA is not convinced they are the ideal solution. What if the lead pilot took a benzodiazepine such as temazepam the night before landing? (Temazepam has a ten- to twelve-hour half-life. Taking a 30-milligram tablet at bedtime is like taking a 15-milligram tablet when you wake up.) What if there were an emergency aboard the shuttle, and the astronauts had to be awakened from a drug-induced sleep? The whole mission might be jeopardized. Since most astronauts experience sleep problems yet their performance is so critical, NASA is now exploring the use of melatonin as a sleep aid.

HOW MELATONIN AIDS SLEEP

Melatonin researchers do not agree on exactly how melatonin helps people sleep. There are two possible mechanisms: (1) it may alter your circadian rhythms, shifting the time that you normally fall asleep to a more desirable time of day; and/or (2) it may have a direct sleep-inducing effect.[25] While my colleagues debate this issue, they agree about the physiological changes that take place when you swallow a tablet: You feel less tense, your reaction time slows, your pulse rate declines, you feel a sense of tranquillity, your body temperature drops, and you begin to feel sleepy. These multiple changes are referred to as "opening the sleep gate." Once the gate is open, it is much easier to fall asleep.

Melatonin's effect on body temperature is one of the keys to its ability to enhance sleep. It has been known since 1835 that the temperature of the human body has a distinct circadian rhythm, rising during the day and falling at night. The daily swing in temperature is only about a degree, but it still has a strong influence on sleep. As a rule, it is easier to fall asleep when your body temperature is falling and to wake up when it is on the rise. Interestingly, you will fall asleep the most quickly and sleep the longest if you turn out the lights while your body temperature is dropping the most rapidly.[26] This fall happens to coincide with the steepest *rise* in your nightly melatonin levels, which takes place somewhere between nine P.M. and twelve A.M., depending on your unique circadian rhythm. If you go to bed at some other point in your melatonin cycle, either earlier or later, your sleep may be neither as restful nor as long.

Until recently, it was thought that the nightly rise in melatonin production and the nightly dip in body temperature were coincidental, that they took place at the same time, but one did not cause the other. Now elaborate studies have shown that melatonin has a *direct* effect on body temperature. Researchers have found that if you take a melatonin tablet during the daytime, when your natural melatonin levels are low and your body temperature is high, it will lower your temperature. Conversely, if you block your melatonin production at night by exposing yourself to very bright light or by taking a melatonin-lowering drug such as a beta-blocker, your body temperature will rise.

THE HOT BATH EFFECT

You can also change your melatonin levels by changing your body temperature. In one study, volunteers sitting in a hot bath in the middle of the day experienced about a two-degree rise in body temperature. Blood samples drawn from them showed an accompanying rise in their melatonin level. Sitting in a lukewarm bath, however, produced no rise in body temperature nor in melatonin level.

This effect may be why taking a hot bath or shower at night helps you fall asleep more quickly: The hot water raises your body temperature, which causes your pineal gland to produce melatonin—perhaps in an effort to maintain a stable temperature. The melatonin causes your temperature to drop back down, swinging open the sleep gate and welcoming you into the land of Nod.[27]

MELATONIN GOES HEAD-TO-HEAD WITH A BENZODIAZEPINE

No investigation into melatonin's sleep-enhancing properties would be complete without comparing the hormone to currently available medications. How does nature's sleeping pill stack up to the competition? In a study now under way at OHSU, volunteers (normal sleepers) are being given either 10 milligrams of melatonin, a placebo, or a commonly prescribed benzodiazepine called temazepam (Restoril). To make the study as naturalistic as possible, the subjects are allowed to sleep in their own homes in their own beds. Just before going to bed, they are given one of the three preparations and are then hooked up to a sophisticated device that monitors their sleep.

The preliminary data from this study shows that melatonin is just as effective as temazepam in reducing the amount of time it takes the subjects to fall asleep. It also extends sleep the same amount of time. But unlike temazepam, melatonin does not delay REM sleep, and therefore it results in a more normal sleep architecture.[28] (See Figures 19 and 20.) Thus melatonin may be less expensive, safer, better tolerated, and less disruptive of normal sleep than this widely prescribed sleep medication. According to a recent review of melatonin, "the clock is ticking for the traditional treatments for insomnia."[29]

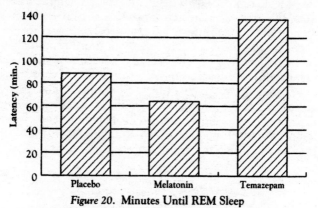

Figure 20. Minutes Until REM Sleep

Subjects who took a sleep medication (temazepam) took much longer to enter their first cycle of REM sleep than subjects who took a placebo or melatonin.

WHOSE SLEEP BENEFITS MOST FROM MELATONIN?

So far, melatonin seems to have a sleep-inducing effect in virtually all volunteers. The current thinking among researchers, however, is that two groups of individuals are most likely to benefit from taking melatonin as a sleep aid: (1) people who produce relatively low amounts of the hormone, and (2) those whose melatonin rhythms are out of phase with their desired sleep schedules. This latter group includes shift workers, jet travelers, people who produce melatonin unusually early or late at night, and those whose melatonin rhythms shift from day to day.

The elderly, however, may benefit most of all. They are likely to have both problems—low levels of melatonin and an altered melatonin rhythm. It is well documented that older people produce less melatonin than younger people. In addition, they start producing melatonin earlier at night, and even more importantly, they *stop* producing it earlier in the morning. When the cycle of melatonin production is shifted to an earlier time of the night, the rhythm is said to be "phase-advanced." Older women as a group may be more phase-advanced than men.[30] As a result, they feel sleepy earlier in the evening and wake up earlier in the morning. Interestingly, surveys show that women go to bed around the same time as men, yet they are likely to wake up earlier in the morning. This could be why so many older women are unhappy with the quality of their sleep—they get less total sleep time.

Older people also show a disruption in the normal stages of sleep. Compared with younger adults, they get less priority sleep (REM and stages III and IV sleep).[31] Benzodiazepines can make matters worse by causing a further reduction in these key stages. Yet the elderly are prescribed these drugs more often than any other age group.

What about the elderly who are good sleepers? How do they differ from those with insomnia? As you may have guessed, they produce more melatonin. A 1994 Israeli study found that elderly people who were good sleepers had significantly higher melatonin levels than those with insomnia.[32] OHSU researchers, too, have found that older people who produce relatively high levels of melatonin sleep longer at night and spend more time dreaming. For the older set, taking melatonin at night may be just as straightforward as taking iron supplements for iron deficiency—it cures what ails them.

What is the best dose of melatonin for older people? It has yet to be determined. The OHSU group has been exploring a wide range of possibilities. On the high end, they've given elderly patients as much as 50 milligrams and have found that that dose actually improves their sleep architecture, helping older people have a more youthful pattern of dreaming.[33] Soon the researchers will know if lower doses produce a similar effect. They already have some indication that the range of effective doses for the elderly may go as low as 0.2 milligrams.[34]

▶ ALZHEIMER'S PATIENTS

Elderly people with Alzheimer's disease tend to have great difficulty sleeping, especially in the later stages of the disease. Caring for them at home can be extremely difficult because of the constant worry that they will wander away in the middle of the night or cause injury to themselves. Surveys have shown that one of the main reasons that Alzheimer's patients are institutionalized is that their caregivers are exhausted by their night duties. Finding an effective sleep aid for Alzheimer's patients would allow more of them to stay at home with the people who know and love them. It could also reduce the $84 billion a year that America pays for the care of institutionalized Alzheimer's patients.

A pilot study conducted at OHSU suggests that melatonin may be a significant part of the solution. Very small amounts of melatonin—0.2 milligrams in a time-release pill—increased the total sleep time of some Alzheimer's patients by as much as two hours—a remarkable improvement for such a low dose. The patients who responded the best were those who had had the most trouble sleeping. A more comprehensive study is now under way, using 0.5 milligrams.

HELPING PEOPLE WHO FALL ASLEEP TOO LATE AT NIGHT

For younger people, one of the most promising uses for melatonin is in helping those whose bodies begin producing melatonin too late at night, a disorder called delayed sleep-phase syndrome. This problem is quite common in teens and young adults—so common, in fact, that it is rarely regarded as a disorder. We tend to accept that young people like to "stay up and party." One reason they have this tendency is that their pineal glands don't begin producing melatonin until relatively late at night. In sleep researchers' jargon, their melatonin rhythm is "phase-delayed" —the opposite of older people, who tend to be phase-advanced.

Some young people are so phase-delayed, however, that it can cause serious problems. In 1994, Japanese researchers reported the case history of an eighteen-year-old man who was plagued with insomnia, fatigue, stomachaches, headaches, and mild depression. His symptoms had become so troubling that he had stopped going to school. But staying at home only compounded his problem: Once he had no reason to get up in the morning, he was free to stay up even later at night. Eventually he was falling asleep at six in the morning and waking up in the late afternoon.

The doctors who evaluated the young man diagnosed him as mildly depressed. But they also noted his peculiar sleep schedule and wondered if normalizing his daily routine would solve some of his emotional problems. Before prescribing an antidepressant, they decided to give him melatonin. Each night at eight o'clock, the young man took 5 milligrams. The very first night he took the hormone, he began having a normal sleep schedule. Most of his psychosomatic symptoms disappeared in a matter of days. The researchers concluded that circadian-rhythm sleep disorders may be far more common in young people than is currently thought, especially in children who have difficulty adjusting to school.

Researchers in Milan, Italy, had equal success when they gave melatonin to seven phase-delayed older patients. Before taking melatonin, these patients would not feel sleepy until three or four in the morning. They were given 5 milligrams of melatonin each evening, somewhere between five and seven P.M.[35] On average, the patients fell asleep two hours earlier than before. They experienced no negative side effects, and their sleep architecture remained normal. When they stopped taking the hormone, all of them returned to their phase-delayed rhythm within a week.[36]

USING MELATONIN TO SUPPLEMENT OTHER MEDICATIONS

Melatonin does not solve everyone's sleep problems. In particular, it may not be effective for people kept awake by moderate to severe pain, marked anxiety, or deep depression. But research is now under way to determine if melatonin added to other medications might provide a safe and effective remedy for these common conditions. For example, OHSU researchers are now conducting a pilot study to see if combining melatonin with a benzodiazepine will help people with anxiety-related sleep problems. Preliminary results suggest that in normal subjects, this combination produces a more restful sleep than benzodiazepines alone.

Other people who might benefit from supplementing their medications with melatonin are those with chronic fatigue syndrome or fibromyalgia, conditions characterized by nonrestorative sleep. Many people with these problems don't produce the expected delta brain wave pattern while they are in deep sleep. Instead, they produce a mixture of delta and alpha waves. (Alpha waves are normally produced only while awake.) This mixed state is called alpha/delta sleep. When alpha waves intrude into deep sleep, they cause a low level of arousal that keeps people from deriving all the benefits from sleep.

Some people with fibromyalgia find that melatonin alone solves their sleep problems. Billie Sahley, Ph.D., the founder of the Pain and Stress Center in San Antonio, has recommended melatonin to a number of patients with this condition. She says, "They take three milligrams at bedtime, and they sleep much better. They also experience less pain." But other people with this condition require additional medications as well. (Amitryptyline plus melatonin is a frequently used combination.)

SLEEP PROBLEMS CAN BE RESOLVED

From talking with sleep researchers, I have learned that most sleep problems can be resolved. But sometimes it takes an expert to pinpoint the cause of the problem and prescribe the right treatment. Diagnosis can be complicated by the fact that insomnia has so many causal factors, including pain, stress, anxiety, age, depression, the side effects of prescription drugs, iron-deficiency anemia, breathing disorders, kidney dysfunction, and diabetes. Sometimes insomnia is caused not by physical or emotional problems but by deeply ingrained sleep habits that can seem very resistant to change.

If you have a severe or long-standing sleep problem, I suggest you consult a sleep specialist. For the name of a qualified sleep clinic near you, write to the National Sleep Foundation, 1367 Connecticut Avenue, N.W., Washington, D.C. 20036.

CHAPTER 9

▼

BACK IN SYNC

Shift work and jet lag are problems unique to human beings. Consider shift work. I know of no animal that shifts its schedule from day to night on a regular basis; animals are either nocturnal (night active) or diurnal (day active). Jet lag is another human invention. Although many animals travel great distances, they have the good sense to migrate north and south, keeping their journeys within one or two time zones. We human beings are the only creatures who routinely shift our work schedules and engage in transmeridian travel, throwing our body clocks out of whack.

One of the latest discoveries to emerge from the research lab is that melatonin is an effective remedy for negative symptoms in both situations. It does two jobs at once: It helps you sleep better, and it resets your body clock, reducing the problems of jet lag and shift work alike.

A CLOSER LOOK AT THE BODY CLOCK

What exactly *is* the body clock, and what does it have to do with melatonin? The term *body clock* refers to a tiny bundle of nerves called the suprachiasmatic nuclei, or SCN,[1] located in the brain directly behind the eyes. The nerve cells of the SCN transmit chemical messages on a regular schedule, approximately twelve hours "on" and twelve hours "off." (The total duration of the cycle is about twenty-five hours.) This built-in rhythm is unique to SCN cells. They persist in it even if they are removed from the body, proving that the rhythm is generated from within. The SCN is believed to be the ultimate source of the body's circadian rhythms.

But there's a problem. The entire body needs to march to the beat of the body clock, yet there is no network of nerves connecting the SCN with all the cells in the body. Somehow the signal has to be conveyed to the rest of the organism. To solve this problem, the SCN signals the pineal gland to produce melatonin that is then dispersed into the circulatory system, a communication network that does, in fact, reach every cell. In essence, melatonin functions as the hands of the body clock.[2]

Here's how the process works in more detail. A set of nerves connects the body clock to the pineal gland. The pineal gland is programmed to produce melatonin only when a chemical signal comes down that pathway. (The signal from the SCN releases a neurotransmitter called norepinephrine, which stimulates pineal cells to produce melatonin. No signal, no norepinephrine; no norepinephrine, no melatonin.) When the body clock is in its twelve-hour "on" phase, the pathway is active and melatonin is produced. When the body clock is in its twelve-hour "off" phase, the pathway is silent and the gland ceases production. Thus melatonin is produced in lockstep with the circadian rhythm of the body clock. The hormone is absorbed into the bloodstream as soon as it is synthesized, sending a signal throughout the body that the SCN is on.

▶ THE BODY CLOCK AND THE SUN

Another matter of timing must be taken care of by the body clock as well. Humans are diurnal creatures. We are programmed to be out and about while the sun is shining and to be home in bed at night. This is why melatonin, the rest-and-recuperate hormone, is produced during the dark hours. But the SCN, by itself, pays no heed to the time of day. It's like a watch that's not adjusted to local time. It may keep perfect time, but it has no built-in relationship to the rising and setting sun.

Somehow the body clock has to be synchronized with the outside world. It gets synchronized by a separate pathway of nerves that leads from the eyes to the body clock. When light from the sun (or some other bright light source) shines in the eyes, a message is sent down the pathway to the body clock, switching it to the "off" phase. When the body clock is off, it sends no signal to the pineal gland, and melatonin is not produced. It is as if the sun reaches into the brain and shuts down melatonin production. About twelve hours later, the body clock turns itself back on, the signal for the pineal gland to resume production. It releases melatonin into the bloodstream, and the circulatory system carries the hormone to the body's trillions of cells. The cells "interpret" this signal as a message of darkness.

I am struck by the simplicity and effectiveness of the body's timekeeping mechanism. The eyes, a central part of the nervous system, gather information about the lighting conditions in the outside world and convey it to the body clock. The body clock sends a chemical message that activates the pineal gland. The pineal gland produces a hormone, melatonin. Melatonin circulates throughout the bloodstream, giving the body information about the time of day. Thus, the role of the pineal gland is to convert a chemical signal (norepinephrine) into a hormone, providing a bridge between the two great information networks of the body, the nervous system and the endocrine system.[3]

► CHANGING THE HANDS
  OF THE BODY CLOCK

Once researchers figured out how the body keeps time, they began to wonder whether we clever humans could somehow intervene in the process. There are several situations in which the body clock fails to conform to the twenty-four-hour cycle. Night shift work and transmeridian travel are two examples. If you work the night shift or fly across time zones, your body clock will adjust eventually, but it may take about a day for each hour your schedule is shifted.

Two quite different modes of intervention came to mind. One would be to expose people to artificial bright light. The light would stand in for the sun, making the body think that the sun was rising or setting at a new time of day. A second strategy would be to give people melatonin. The timekeeping hormone would send a message of darkness, preempting the body's nocturnal production of the hormone.[4] We now have evidence that both of these strategies work, but melatonin offers certain advantages over light therapy. It is less expensive, less time-consuming, and more portable. For these reasons and others, melatonin's ability to reset the body clock has the potential to improve the lives of millions of shift workers and frequent flyers.

THE HIGH COST OF SHIFT WORK

I have done my share of shift work. Because melatonin is produced primarily at night, most of the hundreds of animal experiments I've conducted have taken place in the dead of night. Today, even though I'm a senior researcher with a lab full of competent scientists to conduct the actual experiments, I almost always participate. I hate to miss the camaraderie that develops during those all-nighters. Also, if I observe the experiment as it is being conducted, I've found, I can better interpret the results. If some inconsistency crops up in the data, for example, I can think back to what took place in the lab and perhaps come up with an explanation.

It's not just pinealogists who work the night shift, though. In the United States, approximately 10 percent of all adults have jobs that require them to stay up at odd hours. Between three and five A.M., the sleepiest time of the night, as many as 10 million Americans are hard at work.[5] In Europe, the percentage is even higher, perhaps as much as 15 percent of the adult population.

People vary a great deal in their ability to tolerate shift work. It's been said that in a given group of a hundred shift workers, ten will enjoy working at night and will have no trouble adapting to the schedule; twenty will hate it and will quit as soon as possible; and seventy will have a hard time adapting but will stick with the job for a variety of reasons, including the higher pay. Of the reluctant seventy, a high percentage will be plagued with a disorder called shift maladaptation syndrome. Typical signs of this syndrome are chronic sleep problems, indigestion, ulcers, depression, chronic illness, an increased risk of miscarriage, heart attack, and coronary artery disease. The seriousness of these health problems gives new meaning to the term *graveyard shift*.

Working at cross-purposes to your biological rhythms is harder on your body than it first might appear. Imagine that, tonight, you have to switch your regular schedule to night work. Your scheduled work hours are eleven P.M. to seven A.M. You head off for work at ten-thirty at night, just when your pineal gland is producing a strong surge of melatonin. The hormone signals your heart to slow down, your blood vessels to relax, your body temperature to lower, and your digestion to grind to a halt. You have just entered the Sleep Zone. To fight off a wave of sleepiness, you stop at a fast-food restaurant and gulp down a sixteen-ounce container of coffee, which helps you feel more alert. (Unbeknownst to you, the coffee is inhibiting your production of melatonin.[6]) But your stomach, which has already closed down for the night, resents the hot dark brew, and you feel a bit queasy.

You arrive at work and struggle gamely to stay alert, but at times during the eight-hour shift, particularly around two or three in the morning, you almost fall asleep on your feet. You feel cold, unmotivated. Your reaction time is slow. Your brain feels half asleep. One reason for this slump is that you are producing peak amounts of melatonin.

When the shift ends at seven A.M., you are weary and ready for bed. But your body clock has not had time to shift to the new schedule and is sending a signal to your pineal gland that it's time to *wake up*, shutting down your production of melatonin. As your melatonin level falls, your temperature rises, your pulse quickens, and you feel more alert. The drive home in the bright morning sun makes matters worse by further inhibiting your production of melatonin. Now you are wide awake.

When you arrive home, you're surrounded by dozens of external signs telling you that it's time to wake up, not to go to bed—the morning paper is on the breakfast table; coffee is brewing; the kids are eating their cereal; the hosts on the morning TV news show are wishing you a cheery good day. The whole world seems to be conspiring to keep you awake.

Yet you have to sleep. You eat breakfast and shower, then turn in for the "night." You flop into bed—but sleep does not come. Your heart seems to be racing. Your mind is alert and active. Your hearing seems especially acute. (Does your neighbor *have* to use his gas-powered leaf blower in the morning?) Even though you desperately need to sleep, every cell in your body seems wide awake.

If you stick with your new work schedule, your body clock may or may not adjust to the new routine. Studies show that you have the greatest likelihood of adapting if you are relatively young and happen to be a night owl. If you are thirty or older and function best in the morning hours, you are a poor candidate for shift work and are more likely to suffer from shift maladaptation syndrome.

Even though you continue to show up for work every night, your body clock will remain on strike.

► HELPING SHIFT WORKERS SHIFT

A great deal of effort has gone into finding new therapies and techniques to help shift workers cope. Left to their own devices, many shift workers practice the art of self-medication. At night, they load up on coffee or other stimulants so they can stay awake. In the morning, they wind down by drinking alcohol or taking sleeping pills.

A more promising approach is bright light therapy. Shift workers who are exposed to bright light at the right time of day can shift their biological rhythm so it is in harmony with their work schedule. The bright light substitutes for the sun, convincing their body clock that the sun is shining at night. In a matter of five or six days, they are producing high amounts of melatonin during the day, when they need to sleep, and low amounts at night, when they need to work.

There are two ways that shift workers can increase their light quotient: (1) They can work in a highly illuminated environment, which may require the cooperation of management; or (2) they can purchase a light box and use the device at home. (See Chapter 13.) For maximum benefit, however, workers must avoid bright light during the daytime. They are encouraged to avoid the sunlight or wear very dark glasses or goggles.

Melatonin is a more practical and less costly remedy than light therapy. It, too, resets the body clock, making it the "first clinically viable pharmacological agent that influences the human circadian pacemaker."[7] By sending a message of darkness to the body clock, it causes the body clock to believe the sun is setting in the morning. After about a week of melatonin supplementation, the biological rhythms of many shift workers are more in harmony with their nocturnal schedules. As an added bonus, the signal that melatonin sends to the body clock is so powerful that it overrides the conflicting message from the sun. That means that shift workers can be out in the sun in the daytime and still have their bodies convinced it is night.

▶ NIGHT SHIFT SOLUTIONS

Researchers at Oregon Health Sciences University (OHSU) are now studying melatonin's effects on a group of nurses who work the night shift at a nearby Kaiser Hospital. The nurses work ten-hour days, arriving at work at 9:30 P.M. and leaving at 7:30 A.M. They stay on this schedule for seven days, then have a full week off. (It is called a 7-70 shift.) The nurses take either a small dose of melatonin (0.5 milligrams in an immediate-release format) or a placebo at around nine in the morning, just before they go to sleep. The results are preliminary, but so far, this simple, convenient, and inexpensive treatment has reset the body clocks of a number of nurses who have had difficulty adapting.

Meanwhile, some shift workers have gotten a jump on the researchers and are taking melatonin on their own. Says one of the OHSU researchers, "We have to be careful to screen the participants in our study to make sure they haven't been taking melatonin all along."

I've spoken with a number of shift workers who rely on melatonin to help them adapt. Recently, I interviewed a male nurse who works the night shift in a large hospital in New York. He told me he had read about melatonin in a magazine. He had started taking it to see if it helped him sleep during the day. Normally he would be wired when he came home, so it would take him a long time to settle down. Drinking a couple of beers helped him fall asleep, but most days he would awaken two or three times, partly because of the street noise. Now he takes one milligram of melatonin at nine o'clock in the morning and sleeps seven hours at a stretch. "Taking melatonin is a heck of a lot better than coming home and having a couple of beers.

And it's a deep sleep," he reports. "I don't wake up nearly as often."

JET LAG

You know the symptoms—insomnia, fatigue, irritability, stomach upset, headache, disorientation, and lack of concentration. While you were winging your way across the globe, your body clock was "lagging" behind. You may have been traveling by jet, but your body clock was coming by slow boat or train. Eventually, your body clock will catch up, but it may take a full day or more for each time zone you've crossed.

If you were to fly from San Francisco to Rome, for example, you would be crossing nine time zones. That means that nine days after you arrived, your biological rhythms would be fully adapted to local time. But by then, it would likely be time to turn around and go back home. When your plane touched down in San Francisco, you would be confronted with jet lag all over again, because now your inner clock would be stuck behind in Rome.

As a rule, it's easier to adapt when you fly west. As I mentioned earlier, your body clock actually operates on about a twenty-*five*-hour schedule. Flying west demands that you stretch out your day, going to bed later than you did in your hometown. Your native twenty-five-hour cycle helps you stay up later than normal. Flying east, however, demands that you compress your daily schedule, taking away this built-in advantage.

▶ OLD-FASHIONED REMEDIES

Many travelers rely on sleeping pills to cope with jet lag. But sleeping pills have limited usefulness. Although they help you sleep, they do not adjust your body clock. What they do is send a powerful sleep signal to your brain that simply overwhelms the subtler messages coming from your body clock, allowing you to sleep even though your body clock says that it's the middle of the day. Thus, although the pills alleviate one of the primary symptoms of jet lag—fatigue—they do not address the underlying problem.

In a search for a more natural solution, a number of enterprising people have devised "jet lag diets," complicated dietary regimens that involve eating carbohydrates or proteins at specific times of the day and timing your consumption of caffeine. These diets rely on the fact that eating high-protein food tends to energize you and eating high-carbohydrate food can make you drowsy. Thus manipulating your diet may make it easier for you to fall asleep or stay awake as your new schedule demands. But jet lag diets do not reset your body clock. Like sleeping pills, they treat only the symptoms.

Light therapy is more effective than dietary interventions because light has a direct effect on your body clock. By exposing yourself to bright light at certain times of the day and avoiding light at others, you hasten your body clock's transition to local time. The most effective schedule of light therapy has been worked out by doctors Alfred Lewy and Surge Daan and popularized in a number of jet lag handbooks. These handbooks take into account the number of time zones you've crossed and the direction you've traveled. But drawbacks to this technique include having to arrange your activities around your need for light and darkness. You may also have to pack along a bulky and fragile light box or other lighting device.

▶   A NEW THERAPY FOR JET LAG

Given the drawbacks to these jet lag remedies, it's no wonder that a growing number of frequent flyers are tucking a bottle of melatonin into their carry-on luggage. The person who has been most instrumental in developing a melatonin therapy for jet lag is my longtime colleague Josephine Arendt, Ph.D., professor in the department of biochemistry at the University of Surrey, Guildford, England.[8] The therapy is simple yet effective. The day you arrive at your new destination, you take 5 milligrams of melatonin an hour before bedtime, local time. Melatonin performs two jobs simultaneously—it helps you sleep better, and it speeds up the adjustment of your body clock. Furthermore, it accomplishes both of these ends without inconveniencing you or causing negative side effects. Relieving jet lag is one of melatonin's most straightforward and effective uses.

Several years ago, the recommended strategy was to take melatonin before leaving home. The melatonin adjusted the body clock before and during the flight, allowing people to arrive at their destinations symptom free. This protocol was followed by ten sports physicians and coaches from Italy who were attending the 1990 world karate championships in Mexico. They had stayed in Mexico long enough to become adapted to local time. Before returning home, four of them took melatonin at four o'clock in the afternoon, which corresponded to bedtime in Italy. The remaining six served as controls. When the group arrived in Italy, "the four melatonin volunteers were found to be in perfect mental and physical condition . . . whereas the six controls showed all the classic symptoms of jet lag for 2 to 3 days."[9] (The reason that the current recommendation is to begin treatment upon arrival is that this protocol does not require any elaborate calculations about when to take melatonin.)

Another and larger study produced equally good results. French researchers conducted a jet lag study involving thirty volunteers who were scheduled to fly from the United States to France. One of the criteria for being included in the study was having had difficulty with jet lag in the past. On the day of the flight and for three days thereafter, the volunteers took either a placebo or a tablet that contained 8 milligrams of melatonin. The pills were taken between ten and eleven P.M., French time. The volunteers who took melatonin fared better in every measure tested, including quality of sleep, mood, and work efficiency.[10]

I have been using melatonin to treat jet lag for years, as have many of my colleagues. A recent convert is Peggy Whitson, Ph.D., a researcher at the Medical Sciences Division at the NASA/Johnson Space Center. In her work for NASA, Whitson travels frequently to Russia. Before she learned about melatonin, she would find it difficult to sleep through the night once she arrived. Typically, she would awaken around three A.M. local time and find it hard to get back to sleep. Now she takes melatonin and sleeps very well. "I feel more alert in the afternoon, which is the hardest time to stay awake," she says. "It works great. I'm really impressed."[11]

► FIGHTER JET LAG

During military operations, jet lag can be more than an inconvenience—it can contribute to who wins the war. Sun Tzu, the fourth-century-B.C. tactician who wrote the great Chinese classic *The Art of War*, gave sound advice when he said, "The one who first knows the measures of far and near travel wins—this is the rule of armed struggle."

Never was Sun Tzu's advice more true than during the Persian Gulf War, when the United States had to fight an enemy halfway around the world. Tens of thousands of personnel and thousands of tons of equipment had to be transported as far as six thousand miles, an air bridge that spanned ten time zones. The organization responsible for this massive operation, the Military Airlift Command, was under tremendous pressure to complete the buildup as quickly as possible. Some pilots had to remain awake twenty-four hours at a stretch, subjecting themselves to a dangerous combination of stress, jet lag, long hours, night work, and insufficient sleep.[12]

No one was more aware of the stress being placed on the pilots than Jonathan French, Ph.D., a research physiologist at Brooks Air Force Base in San Antonio. French is assigned to the Sustained Operations Branch, where his job is to "find ways to keep people awake when they'd rather be sleeping and asleep when they'd rather be awake." The biggest problem for crew members, he found, was getting enough sleep. "It's hard to sleep when your body clock is telling you it's noon," says French. "This is especially true on military bases. People are working around the clock. Planes are taking off at all hours. Just because your commanding officer says you have the next eight hours off, that doesn't mean you're going to sleep." Surveys show that at times some of the key flight crew in Operation Desert Storm were so tired, they felt unable to function.

To help the pilots get their much-needed rest, flight surgeons had the authority to prescribe temazepam (Restoril), the only sleep medication currently approved by the air force, albeit with reluctance. Temazepam can cause memory and performance problems. As a precautionary measure, pilots are grounded for twelve hours after taking the drug. According to French, "With benzodiazepines, you're basically intoxicated. It's more than just being sleepy."

French and others are now exploring the possibility of using melatonin as a remedy for jet lag and insomnia. "Based on some of the studies we've done, melatonin may be a very effective sleep aid for the military," he says. "When you take a high dose, you feel like it's two A.M. You're tired and you want to sleep. But if you have to, you can perform. You don't feel drugged. And you're not going to forget what you've done."

In the near future, the air force will be conducting a jet lag study using melatonin. As many as a hundred military personnel who are scheduled to fly to Europe will be given either melatonin tablets or placebos. The volunteers will be studied to see how well they perform various physical and mental tasks and how quickly their body clocks adjust. "I've done preliminary studies," French says, "and some of the results are pretty impressive." Future military operations may go a bit smoother, thanks to melatonin.

CHAPTER 10

▼

A MASTER SEX HORMONE

When I was in graduate school in the early 1960s, I was curious about the newly discovered hormone melatonin, so I went to hear a lecture on the topic given by a fellow medical student. I was not impressed by what I heard—he was able to summarize all that was known about the hormone in ten minutes. I left the lecture hall with one clear thought: "There's no meat on *those* bones."

I doubt if I'd have given melatonin another thought if fate hadn't intervened. As soon as I earned my doctoral degree, I had to fulfill a two-year military requirement, which I was able to do by conducting medical research in the U.S. Army Medical Service Corps. (This was a great relief. My original assignment was to be an artillery officer.) I was assigned to the Army Chemical Center near Baltimore, Maryland, where I joined Dr. Roger Hoffman in the military's search for the "hibernation factor," as I mentioned in Chapter 2.

Hoffman and I wanted to observe the hibernation process in action, so in one of our first experiments we exposed a group of male Syrian hamsters to the conditions known to trigger hibernation—cool temperatures and long periods of darkness. After a few weeks, we took the animals out of their cages and examined them to see if any changes had taken place. One change was patently obvious: The winterlike conditions had shriveled up the hamsters' testes. The change was easy to spot because hamsters have very large gonads for their size, about 5 percent of their body weight. (For the average human male, this would be equivalent to eight-pound testes.) Furthermore, the little rodents seem inordinately proud of their gonads. They will lie in a cage with their testicles pushed to the front, as if to say, "Look at these suckers!" But alas, the month of short days and cool temperatures had robbed the little animals of their pride and joy. Hamsters living in the wild, we found, go through a similar reversal of fortune each winter. When spring comes, their gonads plump up again, and the little animals burst upon the scene in search of potential mates. To insure that young hamsters are born in the late spring, a time of mild climate and abundant food, Nature has found a way to banish thoughts of sex during the fall and winter.

Hoffman and I became curious about how Nature accomplishes this feat. It was our assumption that the winterlike conditions triggered the release of some unidentified hormone that inhibited reproduction. Which hormone was it, and where was it produced? About the same time, Julius Axelrod, Richard Wurtman and other colleagues at the National Institutes of Health had data showing that the pineal gland was more active under conditions of darkness. Hoffman and I made a trek to NIH (which was just down the road) to discuss this new information. From this and other research, we concluded that the pineal gland might be the source of the antigonadal hormone. To test whether this assumption was correct, we decided to remove the pineal glands of male rodents and then place the animals in cool and dark conditions. If the inhibitory hormone was indeed produced by the pineal gland, then those animals without the gland should remain in prime mating condition.

Our first task was to remove the pineal glands from a group of hamsters. It was tricky because the gland is no bigger than the period at the end of this sentence. We had to use an operating microscope to perform the operation. When the animals recovered from the surgery, we put them in the hibernating dens. To have a basis for comparison, we included a group of animals that still had their pineal glands. Then we waited. After about two weeks, Hoffman suggested that we examine the animals. He was like a kid who couldn't wait until Christmas. I persuaded him to hold off a little longer. Finally, after four weeks, we opened the cages and got our first good look at the animals. The difference between the two groups was remarkable. The animals *with* pineal glands had shriveled-up gonads—the expected response to the environmental conditions. But the animals *without* pineal glands were flaunting regulation-size-and-weight testicles. Some substance produced by a little dot of a gland could apparently cause a sixfold difference in the size of the animals' testes.[1]

From that moment on, I was hooked on pineal research. Hibernation no longer interested me, except as it might relate to the pineal gland. Here was brand-new territory to explore. I was experiencing the first stirrings of what would become a lifelong passion.

My excitement propelled me on to the next goal—identifying the actual pineal hormone that inhibited reproduction. Hoffman and I assumed that it was Lerner's newly discovered hormone, melatonin, but we had to demonstrate this in the lab. After many years of frustration, we finally were able to prove that our assumption was correct. Melatonin was indeed the chastity hormone.

THE IMPORTANCE OF SEASONAL REPRODUCTION

This discovery had more significance than it might first appear. Hoffman and I had provided the first clear-cut evidence that the pineal gland performed a useful function in *any* organism. It was not vestigial after all. Furthermore, its primary hormone, melatonin, was crucial for species survival. Without melatonin, animals would no longer reproduce at the optimal time of year.

We modern humans can easily overlook the importance of seasonal reproduction. We have the luxury of giving birth at any time of the year, and our young will survive and thrive. But creatures living in the wild must give birth during a very particular time of the year. The closer they live to the North or South pole, the more critical the timing becomes. For example, a species of Arctic reindeer called the Svaalberg reindeer must bear their young during one particular week of late spring or their fawns will not put on enough fat to survive the next winter. If someone were to remove the pineal glands of these reindeer, they would be inclined to mate whenever the mood struck, and some of their offspring would be born in the dead of winter. Many of these young would die, and the species as a whole could disappear.

How does the pineal gland regulate seasonal breeding? In a remarkably simple and elegant manner. The pineal gland is designed to detect the one reliable indicator of time of year: the number of hours between dusk and dawn. All the other seasonal factors—temperature, rainfall, sunshine, humidity, amount of sunshine—can vary tremendously. For example, meteorological records show that on June 12 in Portland, Oregon, the temperature has ranged from a low of 42 degrees F to a high of 95 degrees F. In some years, June 12 was sunny and bright; in others, dark clouds were hanging over the city. For several years the region suffered from a prolonged drought, and one June Portlanders were mopping up after a catastrophic flood.

But without exception, on every June 12 the sun has risen at 5:21 A.M. and set at 8:59 P.M. It is likely to be keeping this annual appointment long after human beings have passed from the earth. In the infinite wisdom of nature, animals have seized upon this one unchanging factor—the timing of the rising and setting sun—as the basis for their seasonal calendar.

But how do animals monitor the length of the day? As you know, melatonin is produced during conditions of darkness. Thus in the winter, when the night is long, melatonin is produced for a relatively long period of time. In the summer, when the sun sets late and rises early, the increased hours of daylight cut short the nocturnal production of melatonin. Animals "interpret" the amount of time that melatonin is produced as the true sign of time of the year. If melatonin is produced for fourteen hours at a stretch, for example, that signifies winter. If it is produced for only ten hours, it must be summer. The duration of melatonin production influences the animals' reproductive hormones, causing them to be inhibited or released in keeping with the changing seasons.

I am overwhelmed by the beauty of this process. On any given day, the earth's journey around the sun determines the hours of darkness: the pineal gland responds to dark conditions by producing melatonin; the reproductive glands monitor the duration of melatonin production; when melatonin is produced for the right amount of time, mating behavior is triggered. It's a fail-safe, sun-linked method of family planning.

Now we know that this annual cycle of melatonin production sets in motion a host of other seasonal changes in animals as well, including changes in the color and thickness of their coats, the sprouting of antlers, and the annual migration. To everything there is a season—thanks, in part, to melatonin.

▶ HUMANS HAVE SEASONAL RHYTHMS AS WELL

It was many years before researchers realized that melatonin triggers seasonal changes in humans as well. But then, the clues were well hidden. After all, we humans don't gather in herds and migrate each fall. We don't change the color of our hair from winter to summer (at least not without help). We don't appear to be seasonal breeders. So why should we think that our physiology is linked in *any* significant way with the seasons? Maybe we are so intelligent or so highly evolved that we have transcended such mundane matters as time of year.

Not so. If you look very closely, you can see remnants of a seasonal breeding cycle in humans. In Seattle, for example, more twins are conceived in the summer months than in the winter months. According to the investigators, the increased hours of daylight "may stimulate multiple ovulation."[2]

This seasonal effect becomes more pronounced the farther north you go. In northern Finland, which is above the Arctic Circle, there is an eight-week period in the summer in which the sun never sets. During this long period of continuous light, the rate of conception increases significantly.

What triggers this baby boom? Could it be the same process Hoffman and I observed in our hamsters—seasonal changes in melatonin production? To find out, Finnish researchers measured the nocturnal melatonin production of a large group of women from northern Finland in the summer and winter. They found that the women had significantly lower levels of the hormone in the summer months.[3] The increased light at night seems to have inhibited their nocturnal production of melatonin, which, in turn, *increased* their fertility, the very same process that takes place in seasonally breeding animals.

If we were to live in the far north under more primitive conditions, however, we might be true seasonal breeders. Frederick Albert Cook, an American physician and Arctic

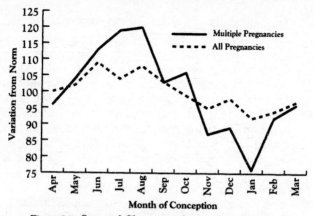

Figure 21. Seasonal Changes in Conception in Finland

explorer, observed this phenomenon while living in an Eskimo village in Greenland in the late 1890s. Native women stopped menstruating in the dark winter months, he learned, and they were not fertile during that period of time. The return of the sun in the spring brought about the resumption of their menstrual cycles and, in both sexes, a resurgence of sexual desire. Cook wrote that the Eskimos exhibited "an intense sexual fury with increasing day lengths."[4]

MELATONIN'S EFFECTS ON FEMALE REPRODUCTION

All well and good, but what effect does melatonin have on reproduction for those of us in more temperate climates? (It is my guess that my story about melatonin causing hamster gonads to shrivel up in the winter caused a few tremors among male readers.) Let's begin by examining what is known about melatonin's role in female reproduction. A number of researchers have shown that a woman's melatonin levels vary over the menstrual cycle. In the most comprehensive study to date, California researchers measured the nocturnal melatonin levels of forty women for two or more menstrual cycles. They found that virtually all the women had a noticeable drop in melatonin right around ovulation. As they neared their menstrual flow, the luteal stage of the menstrual cycle, most women produced significantly more melatonin, almost twice as much as in the first part of the cycle. This is referred to as the "luteal surge."[5]

The drop in melatonin production around the time of ovulation could be significant. It is possible that this decline assists ovulation, in much the same manner that a drop in melatonin level preceding adolescence may usher in puberty. Although this idea has not been confirmed, high levels of melatonin are associated with infertility in women. A study involving female athletes demonstrates this fact. Women who train extensively are more likely to have irregular menstrual cycles or to be amenorrheic, which means they do not menstruate. In 1991 researchers at the University of California at San Diego measured the melatonin levels of eighteen female athletes, eight of whom were amenorrheic. They found that the women

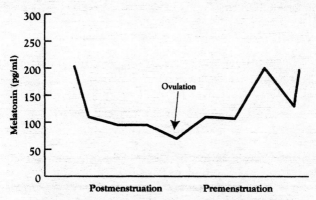

Figure 22. Melatonin Levels over the Menstrual Cycle
Melatonin levels dip at midcycle, which may be involved in triggering ovulation.

who were not menstruating had melatonin levels twice as high as those with normal cycles.[6]

▶ A MELATONIN-BASED CONTRACEPTIVE

Michael Cohen, the developer of the B-Oval contraceptive pill, has had a long-standing interest in melatonin's effects on female reproduction. Noting that a high level of melatonin inhibits ovulation in animals, he wondered if the same was true in women. In a series of pilot studies, he gave women various doses of melatonin. When melatonin was packaged in a slow-release format (extending the amount of time that it remained in the bloodstream), doses as low as 10 milligrams inhibited ovulation in some of the women some of the time. To produce a reliable birth control pill, however, he had to increase the dose of melatonin to 75 milligrams and then combine it with 0.3 milligrams of a progestin called norethisterone (NET).

What is notable about the resulting B-Oval pill is that it is the first oral contraceptive that does *not* contain estrogen. Estrogen-based contraceptives have been linked with a number of potentially life-threatening side effects, including hypertension, blood clots, and an increased risk of breast cancer.[7] Lesser side effects include fluid retention, depression, weight gain, and increased susceptibility to vaginal infection. These pills are not recommended for people with heart disease, liver disease, fibrocystic disease, or fibroid tumors, or women over thirty years of age who smoke.[8]

Because the B-Oval pill does not contain estrogen, it is not likely to have these particular side effects. In fact, it may offer numerous *positive* side effects. For example, Cohen has data showing that his preparation *lowers* blood pressure and cholesterol and causes a substantial improvement in mood.[9] There is also the real possibility that it will lower, not increase, the risk of breast cancer.

► MELATONIN RELIEVES PMS

Premenstrual syndrome (PMS) is a collection of aggravating symptoms that occur just before and during menstruation. Headache, weight gain, carbohydrate craving, insomnia, and irritability are some of the common complaints. Typically, the symptoms get worse as women age. There is some evidence that PMS is associated with low melatonin levels. Studies have shown that women with PMS produce less melatonin than other women, especially in the week before menstruation, when women without this syndrome have a pronounced luteal surge. This happens to be the very time when symptoms of PMS are most evident.[10]

Relief from PMS is one of the many benefits reported by women taking the B-Oval pill. This reaction is so consistent among Cohen's study population that he has developed a melatonin-based treatment for PMS. In his patent application for the new medication, Cohen states, "It has been found that the administration of melatonin to women, preferably during the luteal phase of their cycles, leads to a substantial reduction in, and in some instances, the disappearance of, the symptoms of PMS."[11]

Meanwhile, Dr. Sarafina Corsella, a New York psychia-

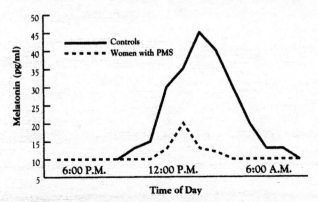

Figure 23. Low Melatonin Levels in Women with PMS

trist who practices holistic medicine, has gotten excellent results treating PMS patients with melatonin. She recommends a dose of 1 or 2 milligrams (taken at night) starting at midcycle and then extending until menstruation. She augments the melatonin with a natural progesterone cream, the amount of progesterone depending on the patient's individual hormonal profile. In some women, she says, the results are phenomenal.[12]

Light therapy has also been shown to reduce the symptoms of PMS, a response that may be due to the light's effects on melatonin production. In one study, women were able to relieve their symptoms of PMS by sitting in front of bright light (2,500 lux) each evening during the week before menstruation. The light extended their nighttime production of melatonin, increasing the amount they produced overall.[13]

▶ WHAT ABOUT MENOPAUSE?

What role, if any, does melatonin play in menopause? There is some indication that melatonin levels decline more rapidly around menopause. In a 1986 study, for example, the melatonin levels of women aged 40 to 59, the menopausal years, was half that of women in the 20 to 39 age bracket. The melatonin levels of men in these two age brackets varied far less.[14]

Follicle-stimulating hormone, or FSH, rises sharply just before menopause. One study has shown that the higher a woman's level of FSH, the lower her levels of melatonin, suggesting once again that melatonin takes a pronounced dip during menopause.[15]

A number of changes occur in a woman's body around the time of menopause that could be related to a sudden drop in melatonin production. Throughout adulthood, for example, the rate of hypertension increases slowly for men, but the incidence for women jumps around age 48, the mean age of menopause.[16] Women have a marked rise in triglycerides and LDL cholesterol just before the onset of menopause.[17] Even more ominous, menopause escalates the risk of coronary artery disease threefold.[18] All of these various conditions have been linked with low levels of melatonin.

In addition, there is anecdotal evidence that melatonin relieves some of the symptoms of menopause, including insomnia and irritability. Cohen has found this to be true in his clinical trials as well and has developed a melatonin-based product to treat menopause. Called M-Oval, the pills contain 75 milligrams of melatonin plus a very small amount of estrogen. "Unlike most hormone replacement therapy," says Cohen, "M-Oval contains no progesterone. Progesterone can have a number of negative effects in women."

The M-Oval pill has the potential to relieve the symptoms of menopause at the same time that it reduces the risk of heart disease and breast cancer. This product is in the second phase of its clinical trials. Preliminary reports are that the women feel better on M-Oval than on traditional hormone replacement therapy (HRT), yet they may get all the benefits associated with HRT, including increased bone density, relief from hot flashes, and improved heart health.

MELATONIN AND THE MALE REPRODUCTIVE SYSTEM

A while ago an article in a men's health magazine suggested that melatonin might compromise a man's virility. The author of the piece mentioned the study I discussed in Chapter 2 about the young man who had such high levels of melatonin that he did not go through puberty until his midtwenties. If high levels of melatonin could delay puberty, the author reasoned, then it must interfere with a man's sex life.

Very little is known about the effects on male sex hormones of high doses of melatonin taken for a prolonged period of time. It is possible that very high doses could have an inhibitory effect. But the levels would have to be much higher than naturally occur during the teenage years, when young men have an abundant supply of both melatonin and testosterone. Another note of reassurance is that more than one study has shown that men who take small doses of melatonin (2 milligrams) show no change in testosterone levels.[19]

What about assertions that melatonin will *improve* one's sex life, claims that are now being made by others? It's a nice thought, but I am sorry to say there is no convincing proof of this contention. But there is some indirect evidence. Michael Cohen reports that women who are on the B-Oval contraceptive pill do not show a diminished sex drive, a side effect associated with estrogen-based contraceptives. This would indicate, however, that melatonin maintains a normal libido, not that it enhances it. And there are some animal studies showing that giving melatonin to aging animals prolongs their sexuality, sometimes quite dramatically. A paper published by an Israeli group in 1995 showed that giving melatonin on a nightly basis to aging rats prevented the age-related decline in testosterone production. In fact, the melatonin-treated rats had almost three times as much testosterone as those not given the hormone.[20]

Another way that melatonin may enhance male sexuality is by increasing the firmness and frequency of erections. Half of all erectile difficulties are believed to be caused by physical, not psychological problems. A common physical cause is constricted arteries. In the same manner that plaque and cholesterol can line the coronary arteries, they can constrict the arteries leading to the penis. If blood cannot flow freely into the organ, the erection is compromised. Melatonin may protect the health of the arteries leading to the penis through its antioxidant and cholesterol-lowering effects.

Finally, melatonin may enhance the motility or forward movement of sperm. Sperm that have low motility are less likely to reach their intended target, the egg. Low sperm motility is associated with low melatonin. In 1988 a group of South African researchers collected blood and semen samples from eighty-five adult men who attended an infertility clinic. The level of melatonin in their blood was found to be closely correlated with the level in their semen. Thus, if a man had high blood levels of melatonin, he was very likely to have high amounts in his seminal fluid. When the samples of semen were divided into groups of high and low melatonin, 63 percent of the sperm in the low-melatonin group had a sluggish forward movement, compared with only 13 percent of the sperm in the high-melatonin group.[21]

CHAPTER 11

▼

MELATONIN AND YOUR MIND

One fact about the pineal gland has captured the imagination of philosophers, mystics, and students of anatomy for centuries—its location in the exact center of the brain. Why does this tiny gland occupy such a privileged and protected position? Early theorists maintained it was due to the fact that the organ was connected with the spiritual side of life.

The first known comments about the pineal gland appeared in the Vedas, ancient religious teachings from India. The gland was portrayed as one of the seven chakras, or centers of vital energy, which are arranged along the central axis of the body. The pineal gland was thought to be the supreme or crown chakra, which is located at the apex of the head.[1] The crown chakra represents the ultimate center of supreme spiritual force and has been referred to as the "gateway to perfect rest and harmony."

A third-century B.C. Greek physician, Herophilus, described the gland as a sphincter that controlled the flow of "animal spirits" (*pneuma psychikon*) between the ventricles (cavities) of the brain and the supposedly hollow nerves. René Descartes, the seventeenth-century mathematician and philosopher, is often credited with calling the pineal gland "the seat of the soul." His exact words, which appear in his *Treatise of Man*, are less eloquent: "there is a small gland in the brain called the pineal in which the soul exercises its function more particularly than in any other part."

In the mid-1700s an Italian student of anatomy named Giovanni Morgagni dissected the brains of a large number of cadavers and noted that people reported to have been "disordered in their minds" had abnormal-looking pineal glands. The glands were filled with calcium deposits and appeared atrophied and nonfunctional. Scholars in the 1800s made the same observation, leading to the assumption that madness is linked with an abnormal pineal gland.

Psychiatrist Mark Altschule, M.D., of McLean Hospital in Boston, was one of the first researchers to act on this assumption. In the 1940s he and a student, Julian Kitay, M.D., began assembling all the known pineal research from around the world, ultimately collecting more than eighteen hundred scientific papers from thirty-eight international libraries. Seventeen of those papers described studies in which physicians had treated schizophrenics with pineal extracts. Altschule was drawn to these particular studies for two reasons—he was a psychiatrist, and his wife suffered from schizophrenia. In the 1950s he injected pineal extracts into a number of schizophrenic patients and is rumored to have treated his wife as well. He reported a number of successes, but his methodology did not satisfy the scientific community causing his findings to be largely ignored.

Later—once melatonin was isolated, identified, and synthesized—researchers began injecting the hormone itself into human volunteers. A common observation was that the hormone made people feel relaxed, calm, tranquil, and sometimes euphoric—hearkening back to the ancient Indian belief that the gland is the "gateway to perfect rest and harmony."

Today researchers are exploring melatonin's potential to treat a wide number of psychological conditions, including depression, bipolar disorder (manic depression), seasonal affective disorder (SAD), schizophrenia, alcoholism, and autism. In the pages that follow I will bring you up to date on some of the most promising findings.

DEPRESSION

As we have seen, one of the surprising findings to emerge from the clinical trial of the B-Oval contraceptive pill (which contains 75 milligrams of melatonin) is that the women taking the medication have an improved mood. According to Michael Cohen, "We do extensive testing of the women, both their physical and mental state. We have found that the women taking B-Oval have many fewer complaints about daily life than they did before taking the pill. Some even report a mild euphoria."

What other evidence suggests that melatonin has an antidepressant effect? One indirect piece of data is that people suffering from some kinds of depression have low melatonin levels. This connection was documented in the late 1970s and early 1980s by a group of Swedish psychiatrists, including Lennart Wetterberg, M.D., from the Karolinska Institute in Stockholm.[2]

More recently, a group of American psychiatrists from the University of Texas Medical Branch at Galveston learned that depressed children may have low melatonin levels as well. In 1987 the researchers measured the hormone levels of a group of depressed boys who were between the ages of 9 and 15. The boys had a third less melatonin than nondepressed boys of similar age and body weight.[3]

Swedish researcher Johan Beck-Friis, M.D., has suggested that traumatic events early in life could cause low melatonin levels. In one of his studies, he noted that depressed adults who were separated from a parent before the age of 17, whether by death or divorce, had very low levels of melatonin—in some cases below the level of detection. The production of melatonin, he conjectured, "could be influenced by strong emotional experiences during critical life phases before the completion of puberty."[4]

This notion is not as far-fetched as it may seem. New evidence suggests that traumatic experiences have the potential to alter the physical structure of the brain. People who have been subjected to extraordinary levels of stress, whether through warfare or abusive parents, have been found to have less tissue mass in key areas of the brain.[5] Cortisol, a stress hormone, may contribute to this physical deterioration. (This hypothesis has been shown to hold true in animals.) Prolonged stress in childhood could also damage the structures of the brain involved in the production of melatonin.

▶ SUICIDE VICTIMS

Studies have shown that most people who commit suicide were suffering from untreated or untreatable depression. Did they have low melatonin levels as well? Dr. Michael Stanley at Columbia University believes the answer is yes. He measured melatonin levels in the pineal glands of nineteen suicide victims and nineteen people who died from other causes. So that the two groups would be as similar as possible, the control group consisted of people who had died suddenly or violently, such as from automobile accidents or gunshot wounds. The groups were matched for age and time of death as well. The results showed that the suicide victims had far less melatonin in their pineal glands than the controls. The difference was especially striking when the deaths occurred at night, the time when melatonin is being actively produced.[6]

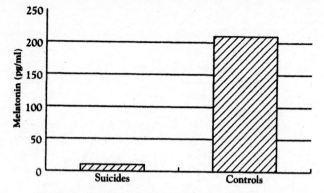

Figure 24. Pineal Melatonin in Suicides and Controls
(10 p.m.–6 a.m.)

▶ WILL STIMULATING MELATONIN PRODUCTION RELIEVE DEPRESSION?

Can depression be relieved by enhancing melatonin levels? This area of research is still in its infancy, but three lines of evidence suggest that it can: (1) Some antidepressants increase melatonin levels; (2) some drugs that increase melatonin levels relieve depression; (3) taking melatonin itself has improved the mood of some people.

One family of antidepressant drugs known to increase nocturnal melatonin is the MAO inhibitors. (Brand names include Marplan, Nardil, and Parnate.) In one study, healthy nondepressed volunteers were given a dose of Parnate during the daytime when their melatonin levels were naturally low. The Parnate caused significantly higher melatonin levels during the next few hours.[7] Other antidepressants that stimulate melatonin production include desipramine (Norpramin and Pertofrane) and fluvoxamine (Luvox). Lithium, a drug commonly prescribed for bipolar disorder, is yet another melatonin enhancer.[8]

Of course, the fact that some antidepressants raise melatonin levels is no proof that stimulating melatonin production relieves depression. It is possible that the increase in melatonin levels is a mere side effect of the drugs. (As a parallel example, one side effect of some antidepressants is a rapid pulse, but no one would suggest that the rapid pulse is responsible for relieving the depression; those two phenomena are merely coincidental.)

Some findings, however, suggest that stimulating melatonin production *does* relieve depression. French researchers recently studied the antidepressant effects of a natural substance called destyr gamma endorphin (DTγE), which causes a significant increase in melatonin levels. In a double-blind experiment, twenty depressed patients were randomly selected to receive either a nightly dose of DTγE or a placebo. Eight of the ten patients who received DTγE felt remarkably better in only five days, which is an unusually fast response to an antidepressant drug. The placebo, on the other hand, had little effect. According to the researchers, these findings demonstrate "a significant and rapid antidepressant activity of destyr gamma endorphin that is devoid of side effects."[9]

A different group of French researchers got equally positive results when they gave depressed patients a nightly dose of another compound known to stimulate melatonin—5-methoxypsoralen, or 5 MOP. As in the DTγE study, the patients receiving 5 MOP experienced a dramatic relief from depression in five days, with no negative side effects.[10]

Depression has also been relieved by taking tryptophan, the amino acid from which melatonin is derived. Taking tryptophan has been shown to increase melatonin levels.[11] In a number of studies involving tryptophan, the relief of depression corresponded with an increase in melatonin production.[12]

In recent years it has been discovered that Saint-John's-wort (*Hypericum*), a common groundcover plant, raises melatonin levels.[13] Saint-John's-wort has been used as a folk remedy for depression for more than two thousand years. Rigorous scientific studies have shown that the herb does indeed have a significant antidepressant effect, yet another substance that relieves depression and also stimulates melatonin production.

▶ DOES TAKING MELATONIN ITSELF RELIEVE DE-PRESSION?

Other than preliminary results from the B-Oval study, is there any evidence that melatonin itself has an effect on depression? One of the first indications that it might came from a 1971 study in which Ferdinando Anton-Tay and colleagues injected five volunteers with large amounts of melatonin.[14] According to their report, "fifteen to twenty minutes later, the subjects fell asleep. They were easily awakened 45 minutes later. At the end of the experiment all the subjects mentioned a sensation of well-being and moderate elation."[15] Two other studies, both conducted in the 1970s, showed that melatonin produced feelings of "contentment and improved mood."[16]

In a more recent study, volunteers who took 5 milligrams of melatonin to relieve jet lag reported an enhanced sense of well-being.[17]

Today pharmaceutical companies are investing billions of dollars in researching the antidepressant properties of melatonin's close cousin, serotonin, the neurotransmitter that is enhanced by drugs such as Prozac and Zoloft. In some respects, melatonin is a more logical candidate as a treatment for depression. Serotonin has difficulty crossing the blood-brain barrier. Therefore, to increase the activity of serotonin in the brain, pharmacologists have to concoct drugs that block the enzymatic destruction of the compound or prevent it from being reabsorbed by neurons. But to increase melatonin levels in your brain, all you have to do is take melatonin. Given the preliminary evidence that melatonin may enhance mood in some people, coupled with its apparent lack of toxicity and negative side effects, it is reasonable to suggest that a few million dollars might be diverted to exploring the antidepressant potential of melatonin.

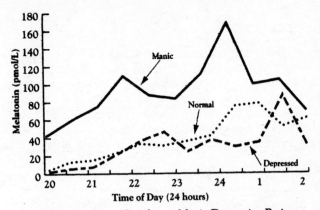

Figure 25. Melatonin Levels in a Manic-Depressive Patient

MANIC DEPRESSION

People who suffer from manic depression, or bipolar mood disorder, are troubled by mood swings that can career from euphoria to despondency. There is some evidence that their melatonin levels go along on the roller-coaster ride, peaking during periods of mania and plummeting during periods of depression. In 1979, for example, Alfred A. Lewy, a psychiatrist at the Oregon Health Sciences University in Portland, and his colleagues observed that bipolar patients had elevated melatonin levels when they were manic and reduced levels when they were depressed. Canadian psychiatrists provided further insight by measuring the melatonin levels of one patient in all three phases of the illness. They drew blood samples from the twenty-nine-year-old woman at three separate occasions: when she was manic, when she was depressed, and when she was feeling normal. They found she was producing more than twice as much melatonin when she was manic than when she was depressed. When she was symptom free, she had normal amounts of the hormone.[18] In this instance, there was a clear correlation between melatonin levels and mood.

SCHIZOPHRENIA

A study of people whose pineal glands had been removed provides further evidence of a link between a healthy pineal gland and a healthy state of mind. After recovering from surgery, the patients were plagued with recurrent symptoms of "depression, anxiety, hypersomnia [excessive sleepiness], headache . . . migraine, auditory illusions, and hallucinations."[19] The fact that pinealectomy can cause visual and auditory hallucinations is of particular interest to those studying a possible connection between low melatonin and schizophrenia.

Indeed, a number of studies have shown that people with schizophrenia have unusually low levels of melatonin. In 1992 I collaborated on a study designed to compare the melatonin levels of a group of drug-free paranoid schizophrenics (a subgroup of schizophrenics) with a group of healthy people of similar ages. We found that the schizophrenics were producing far less melatonin than the control group, as you can see in Figure 26.[20]

To my knowledge, no one has given melatonin itself to schizophrenics to see if it relieves any of their symptoms,

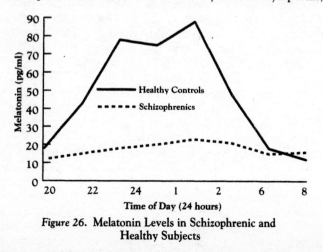

Figure 26. Melatonin Levels in Schizophrenic and Healthy Subjects

but such a study has ample justification. Even if the hormone did not improve the mental state of the patients, it might relieve some of the problems commonly associated with the disease, such as sleep difficulties and a weakened immune system.

CHRONIC PAIN

In 1986 a group of Swedish researchers became interested in the fact that depressed people and chronic pain sufferers have many similarities in their brain chemicals and hormone levels.[21] Would chronic pain sufferers also have low levels of melatonin? As hypothesized, they found that the chronic pain sufferers in their study had low levels of melatonin compared with the controls. Patients with nerve-related pain had the lowest levels of all.[22]

What is most intriguing to me about the relationship between melatonin and chronic pain is that melatonin has potent analgesic properties, suggesting a cause-and-effect relationship between low melatonin levels and pain. A group of researchers from the University of California became interested in the possible pain-relieving properties of melatonin when they noted that many animals are less sensitive to pain at night. This is true for both nocturnal and diurnal animals. In one experiment, they placed mice on a very warm surface and observed how long it took them to show signs of discomfort. It took an average of 62 seconds in the daytime but 110 seconds at night, indicating that the mice had a higher tolerance for pain at night. Other studies had shown that mice are most tolerant of pain shortly after midnight, which is when they have the highest levels of melatonin.

The California researchers' next step was to give rodents varying amounts of melatonin to see if added amounts of the hormone increased their pain tolerance. They found that the more melatonin they gave the rodents, the longer they were willing to stay on the hot surface. At the highest dose (90 milligrams per kilogram) of melatonin, the mice tolerated moderate pain three times as long as they did without melatonin. In fact, dose per dose, melatonin was almost as effective at relieving pain as morphine.[23]

A group of researchers from Canada have explored the relationship between aging, melatonin, and pain. In an initial study, they found that young mice stayed on a hot surface for an average of 46 seconds before showing discomfort, but a group of old mice started licking their feet after only 25 seconds. Were the older mice more sensitive to pain because they had lost their youthful supply of melatonin?

To find out, they injected a group of old mice with melatonin, giving them the melatonin levels of younger animals. The rejuvenated rodents now stayed on the hot surface for 40 seconds, almost as long as young mice. Next, they injected young rodents with a melatonin-lowering drug to see if depriving them of their melatonin supply decreased their tolerance for pain. As expected, the melatonin-deficient young mice became much more sensitive to pain.[24] Taken together, these studies indicate a direct relationship between tolerance for pain and the amount of melatonin circulating in the bloodstream.

Does melatonin have similar analgesic properties in humans? One indication that it might is that the pain threshold in humans has a circadian rhythm, just like that of the rodents. And like the rodents, we are most tolerant of pain when our melatonin levels are highest—in the very early hours of the morning.[25] Hospital records show that patients make the fewest requests for pain medications between midnight and four A.M., which is when their melatonin levels peak. Finally, a number of clinicians around the country have prescribed melatonin for patients with chronic pain and noted significant nighttime relief.

If melatonin, or a melatonin-like substance, could be developed into an effective treatment for pain, it would prove a godsend for millions of people. Forty-four percent of the chronic pain sufferers surveyed in a Louis Harris poll said they were unhappy with the pain medications currently available to them.[26] They were leery of taking over-the-counter medications because of potential side effects, and they were reluctant to take prescription pain-killers because they were afraid they might prove addictive. Melatonin might offer a safe, inexpensive, and effective alternative. It is not addictive, and unlike other pain-killers, it does not cause sleep disturbance or stomach irritation. Melatonin is especially well suited for nighttime pain relief because of its sleep-inducing effects. For daytime use, caffeine could be added to counteract drowsiness.

Pharmaceutical companies are currently developing analogues of melatonin—molecular look-alikes—that do not cause drowsiness or alter the body's circadian rhythms. These compounds could form the basis for a new and improved family of pain-relievers. A more immediate solution for chronic pain sufferers may be to combine melatonin with prescription or over-the-counter pain medications, potentially increasing their effectiveness and diminishing their negative side effects.

ALCOHOLISM

In 1978, Lennart Wetterberg in Sweden measured the melatonin levels of twenty-five consecutive patients who were admitted to a hospital emergency room. Eleven of the patients, he found, had noticeably low levels of melatonin. Upon further investigation, it was discovered that all of these eleven patients had a history of alcoholism.

Interestingly, their use of alcohol varied greatly. Some had been intoxicated when they were admitted to the hospital; some had not had an alcoholic drink in at least three weeks; and others had been abstinent for years. Nevertheless, all eleven had noticeably low levels of melatonin. Wetterberg commented, "It is clear that further studies of the relationship between low melatonin and alcohol abuse are warranted."[27]

In 1992, Wetterberg himself conducted just such an inquiry. This time he collaborated with a group of researchers from the United States who surveyed the melatonin levels of nineteen former alcoholics who were outpatients at a VA medical center in California. The patients had been abstinent for a period of a month to as long as ten years. All refrained from drinking alcohol for the duration of the six-month study. (Their abstinence was confirmed by clinical monitoring.) As in Wetterberg's original study, the former alcoholics were producing much less melatonin than members of a control group who did not have a history of alcoholism.

Why would alcoholics who have been abstinent for years have low melatonin levels? No one knows. But Wetterberg has suggested that chronic use of alcohol might permanently alter the body's ability to produce melatonin.[28] If that is so, then melatonin—a natural substance with no potential for addiction—may be an ideal aid for recovering alcoholics, who often have persistent sleep problems.

SEASONAL AFFECTIVE DISORDER (SAD)

Seasonal depression is known by many names, including atypical depression, seasonal affective disorder (SAD), and the winter blues. For simplicity's sake, I will use the acronym SAD. SAD is much more common than was believed twenty years ago. Norman Rosenthal, a SAD researcher and expert from the National Institutes of Health, estimates that 35 million Americans suffer from winter depression and that as many as 10 million may have severe cases of the syndrome.[29] Three times more women than men suffer from SAD, although no one is quite sure why. It is much more common in people living in the northern and southern latitudes than in those living closer to the equator. For example, SAD affects 10,000 out of every 100,000 people in Minnesota, New York, and Washington State, but only 6 out of every 100,000 people in Florida, Arizona, and Louisiana.[30]

Many of the symptoms of SAD are quite different from the symptoms of nonseasonal depression. People with nonseasonal depression tend to complain of a lack of appetite, insomnia, low self-esteem, and feelings of helplessness or hopelessness. SAD sufferers have a different litany of woes. They are troubled by sleepiness, low energy, social withdrawal, and *increased* appetite—especially for sweets and other carbohydrates.

If you stop to think about it, the symptoms of SAD sound a lot like those of hibernation. Hibernating animals stock up on food in the fall and then climb into a dark hole and sleep out the winter. It doesn't take too much imagination to reframe these behaviors as carbohydrate craving, fatigue, and social withdrawal.

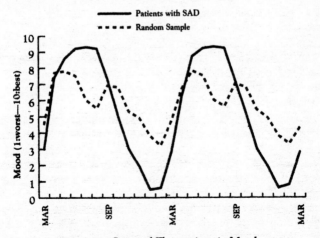

Figure 27. Seasonal Fluctuations in Mood

▶ SAD BUT TRUE

In addition to the millions of people who have bona fide
SAD, many more people have "subsyndromal" SAD, a
milder version of the affliction. In fact, two recent studies
suggest that the majority of the population, including children, feel somewhat blue in the fall and winter. In one of
the studies, more than two thousand parents completed a
questionnaire about the wintertime behavior of their children. Forty-eight percent of the parents said their children
showed one or more signs of winter depression. The most
common was "eats more," followed by "sleeps more,"
"seems irritable," "seems sad," and "withdraws from family
and friends."[31]

   The graph in Figure 27 compares seasonal mood swings
in a random sample of the population compared with patients diagnosed with seasonal affective disorder. As you
can see, we may all be a little bit SAD.

▶ MELATONIN'S ROLE IN SAD

What does SAD have to do with melatonin? There is
some evidence that the hormone might be responsible for
at least one symptom of SAD—increased sleepiness. In
1990, Thomas A. Wehr, a researcher at the National Institutes of Health, subjected eight healthy young men to
lighting conditions that mimicked seasonal changes in day
length.[32] The men spent one week in summer lighting
conditions—sixteen hours of light and eight hours of dark.
Then for the next four weeks, the lights were turned off at
six P.M., plunging the men into the depths of winter. During the long winter nights, they produced melatonin for
an average of two hours longer. But they stayed in bed
three hours longer, akin to a minihibernation.[33]

▶ DON'T BLAME YOUR WINTER WEIGHT GAIN
   ON MELATONIN

Is melatonin responsible for the weight gain that accompanies SAD? It doesn't appear so. Animals that have been injected with melatonin either gain weight or *lose* weight, depending on the species and breed. (For example, Siberian hamsters lose weight, but Syrian hamsters gain weight.) In humans, melatonin appears to speed up our metabolism, making us more efficient calorie-burners. We think this is so because people with SAD have *higher* resting metabolic rates than people without SAD. When SAD patients are exposed to bright light, their melatonin levels go down, as does their metabolic rate, the opposite of what one would expect.

Yet, despite the fact that people with SAD appear to burn calories faster than people without it, they still manage to gain weight in the winter. How can this be? Perhaps their appetite increases enough to offset the faster rate. For example, if you had a higher metabolic rate in the winter, burning, say, 200 additional calories each day, you would expect to lose weight. But if you also had such a hearty appetite that you ate 400 *extra* calories each day, you would have a net gain of 200 calories. Over the span of several months, you could easily gain five to ten pounds. We believe this is what causes many people with SAD to gain weight.

Why do people with SAD want to eat more in the winter? The explanation may be that they have low levels of serotonin, which has a direct effect on appetite.[34] Antidepressant drugs such as Prozac and Zoloft raise the level of serotonin in the brain and have a tendency to suppress the appetite; in fact, many people lose weight on these drugs. Another way to raise your serotonin level is to undergo light therapy. In one study, every patient who was treated with bright light had increased levels of serotonin.[35] Light therapy also tends to decrease appetite. For one hour each day, thirty-six people with SAD sat in front of a specially designed light box (2,500 lux). At the end of two weeks, they were eating 50 percent fewer carbohydrates during the second half of the day than they had before therapy. In another study, ten patients with SAD were treated with nine days of phototherapy. During this period they lost an average of almost two pounds, even though none of them were trying to diet.[36]

Correspondingly, low serotonin levels are associated with carbohydrate craving. It could be that the levels of light present in the winter are insufficient to raise serotonin levels in people susceptible to SAD. This deficiency of serotonin causes them to overeat and gain extra weight. Whether or not this is the precise mechanism involved, the evidence is convincing that getting more light in the winter will decrease your appetite and keep you from gaining weight.

▶ MELATONIN AND SEASONAL SADNESS

The most bothersome symptoms for many people with SAD are low spirits and lack of motivation. For as much as five or six months of the year, SAD sufferers have little zest for life. When spring comes, it is as if a switch is thrown, and they greet the world with new optimism. For these individuals, there seems to be a direct link between hours of sunlight and mood.

This phenomenon was dramatically illustrated in the seasonal lighting study mentioned earlier in this chapter. One of the men became deeply depressed after living for only five days in the winter lighting environment (lights off at six P.M.), even though he had had no previous history of depression. The researchers even had some concern that he might become suicidal, and he was excused from the experiment. Fortunately, his depression lifted as soon as he returned to normal life and was able to lengthen his light exposure. For him, the number of hours of daylight was literally a matter of life or death.

▶ LIGHT THERAPY RELIEVES SEVERE SYMPTOMS OF SAD

A man who has spent many years exploring the biological link between light, moods, and melatonin is Alfred A. Lewy. Lewy first became interested in seasonal depression in the late 1970s while working at the National Institutes of Health. At the time, he had a sixty-three-year-old patient, an engineer, with pronounced mood swings. When depressed, the patient was withdrawn, self-critical, and anxious; he lost his enthusiasm for his normal activities and dreaded going to work. When his depression lifted, he felt better than well—he was filled with energy and needed few hours of sleep.

His would appear to be a typical case of bipolar mood disorder or manic depression, except that the man's mood swings were precisely linked with the seasons. Each year he would begin to feel glum around mid-July. He would remain depressed for the next thirty weeks or so. Around January or February, as the day length began to increase, his depression would lift, and he would feel high spirited until midsummer. He had been to a number of psychiatrists who treated him with the standard medications, including antidepressants and lithium, but he could not tolerate their side effects. Besides, he was convinced there was a more fundamental cure for his mood swings, one that uncoupled the link between the seasons and his sanity.

Fortunately for Lewy, this particular patient was not only an engineer but a bit of an obsessive-compulsive and had been keeping a detailed record of his mood swings for the previous fourteen years. The diary showed an unmistakable correlation between mood and time of year. Lewy hypothesized that exposing him to artificial bright light in the midst of one of his seasonal slumps might trick his body into thinking winter was over, causing his depression to lift spontaneously.

In December 1980, when the patient was mired in depression, Lewy put him on an intensive schedule of light therapy. Each day the man sat in front of a bright light (2,000 lux) for three hours in the early morning and three hours in the early evening, in effect transforming the bleak Washington, D.C., winter into spring. The man's depressive symptoms began to remit in just four days. By the tenth day he felt well.[37]

▶ GLAD CURES SAD

Today tens of thousands of people have learned that the antidote to SAD is GLAD—good light of adequate duration. (You can blame researcher Charles P. Maurizi, M.D., for this new acronym.) The precise mechanism by which light therapy relieves winter depression, however, is much debated. Lewy's explanation is that people with seasonal depression have a "phase-delayed" melatonin rhythm, which means that they start producing melatonin later at night than most people. This throws their circadian rhythms out of whack, making them feel tired and depressed. Exposure to bright light in the morning hours advances the onset of melatonin production to a more normal schedule. A number of studies support Lewy's theory, showing that morning light is more effective than evening light in relieving symptoms of SAD.

An alternative explanation has to do with light's effect on serotonin, not melatonin. It is by raising serotonin levels, in this theory, that light relieves depressive symptoms; any effect on melatonin production is merely incidental. Proponents of this theory argue that bright light at any time of day has been shown to improve the mood of people with seasonal depression, casting doubts on the phase-delay theory.

It may be decades before we understand all the complexities of the intricate dance between serotonin and melatonin, but at this point most experts in the field agree that bright light is a safe and effective therapy for SAD. People who pass the dark days of winter slumped on the couch in between trips to the refrigerator can get relief in as little as three days by increasing their exposure to light. Spending an extra hour out of doors, sitting in front of a specially designed light box, or wearing a new high-tech "light visor" may be all they need to defeat SAD. Meanwhile, Lewy and his colleagues at OHSU are investigating whether taking melatonin at a prescribed time of day can also take the blues out of winter.

CHAPTER 12

▼

THE GREAT ANTI-AGING
EXPERIMENT

Have you not a moist eye, a dry hand, a yellow cheek, a
white beard, a decreasing leg, an increasing belly? Is not
your voice broken, your wind short, your chin double,
your wit single, and every part about you blasted with
antiquity?

Shakespeare, *King Henry IV*

In November 1985, Georges Maestroni and two of his
colleagues began an animal study that would provide the
first convincing evidence of melatonin's ability to extend
life.[1] The experiment involved twenty nineteen-month-
old mice. The researchers divided the mice into two
groups and housed them in identical cages. The animals
were fed the same diet and were exposed to the same
environmental conditions. The only difference was that
each evening ten of the mice were given a trace amount of
melatonin in their drinking water. At this advanced stage
of their life, the mice would be producing little melatonin
on their own. In effect, they were being put on melatonin
replacement therapy.

Five months into the study the researchers observed
what they called an astonishing difference between the

two groups of rodents. The mice that had been drinking plain water were showing the expected signs of aging—they had lost weight, slowed down their pace, begun to sit in a characteristic humped posture, and developed dry patchy fur; they looked like mice that were ready to die. Meanwhile, the melatonin mice were glossy and plump and cavorting around their cages like the octogenarians in the movie *Cocoon*.

The real story, however, unfolded a month later when the mice that were drinking plain water began to die one by one, right on schedule, while the melatonin-treated mice continued to thrive. When the last mouse had died, the researchers discovered that the average survival time of the water-drinking mice was 752 days, typical for this strain of mouse, but the mice that had been given the melatonin nightcaps had lived an average of 931 days—a 20 percent increase in lifespan.[2]

IMPROVING THE QUALITY OF LIFE IN OLD AGE

What would happen if you and I were to take a little melatonin every night? Would we live to be a hundred years old or more? Would we be out on the golf course practicing our approach shots while our few surviving peers were being spoon-fed pabulum in nursing homes?

So far in this book, I've talked very little about melatonin's life-*extending* potential. Instead, my focus has been on its life-*enhancing* properties. To refresh your memory, here's a brief summary of melatonin's potential to improve the quality of life as we age:

1. By scavenging free radicals, melatonin may prevent or reduce the severity of a host of diseases, including cancer, Alzheimer's, arthritis, Parkinson's, and ulcers.

2. By counteracting the effects of aging on the immune system, melatonin may give us added protection against cancer, viruses, bacteria, and parasites. The specter of thousands of old people dying each winter from an ordinary flu virus could become a thing of the past.

3. By giving us a more youthful pattern of sleep, melatonin would allow us to derive maximum benefit from the nightly cycle of rest and repair.

4. By taking a small nightly dose of melatonin, we should be able to stabilize our circadian rhythms, helping to counteract an aging body clock. This, in turn, would help keep all our biological rhythms in tune.

5. Melatonin supplementation may result in a healthier cardiovascular system. Because of its free-radical-scavenging ability and direct heart-protective effects, melatonin might lower blood pressure, cholesterol, and reduce the risk of coronary heart disease.

The question that concerns us in this chapter is whether taking melatonin will allow us to live not just *better* but *longer*. The only way to know with certainty would be to conduct a human longevity study similar to Maestroni's mouse experiment, one in which half the people took melatonin and the other half placebos. Unfortunately, the cost of such a study would be astronomical. Human beings are so genetically diverse that tens of thousands of people would have to be enrolled in the study to get meaningful results. Furthermore, we are such a long-lived species that the study would have to run a minimum of fifty years. Many of us would be in our graves before the findings were announced.

Lacking a definitive clinical trial, the only way to find out if melatonin can extend human life is to weigh the indirect evidence: What can we glean from animal longevity studies such as the Maestroni experiment? What do we know about long-lived people? How does melatonin research mesh with our understanding of the biology of aging? In this chapter I will take you on just such a fact-finding expedition.

WHY DO WE AGE?

The less that is known about a given medical topic, it has been said, the more theories abound. This maxim certainly holds true for aging. Scores of fundamental questions about aging have yet to be resolved, and theories of aging are equally numerous. For example, some theorists maintain that our cells are programmed to divide a finite number of times; once a cell has exhausted its allotment, it must perish. Death occurs when we have lost a significant number of vital cells. Others theorists focus on the immune system, maintaining that a gradual loss of immunity makes us vulnerable to attack from within and without. Still others suggest that a key factor in the aging process is a breakdown of the body's internal timing mechanisms. Once our biological rhythms falter, the body can no longer function in an efficient manner. We're like antique sports cars badly in need of a tune-up, prone to breaking down by the side of the road.

What is interesting about these three proposed mechanisms of aging is that melatonin supplementation could influence all but one—the finite replication of cells. Melatonin therapy has been shown to preserve the immune function of aging animals and to regulate the biological rhythms of both animals and humans.

There is a fourth theory of aging, however, that has more adherents than the first three combined: unrepaired cell damage. According to this theory, we age because too many of our cells become damaged and do not get repaired. Gerontologists argue about the specific nature of the damage: Is it cross-linking of proteins? Damage to cell membranes? Damage to nuclear DNA? Damage to mitochondrial DNA? But most of them agree that cumulative wear and tear on our vital tissues is the underlying cause of aging. This gradual erosion deprives us of neurons, allows cells to become malignant, weakens the heart muscle, clogs our arteries, destroys the energy-producing parts of cells, and reduces our number of viable immune cells.

There is also a growing consensus as to the primary cause of cell damage—free radicals.[3] This idea was first formulated in 1954 by Denham Harman, M.D.[4] At the time he advanced it, Harman's idea was given little credence. Skeptics noted that if free-radical damage did indeed underlie the aging process, then researchers should be able to extend the life span of animals by giving them antioxidant supplements. But antioxidants did not appear to have that effect. They prevented a number of degenerative diseases and allowed a higher percentage of animals to reach old age, but the animals set no longevity records.

DYING LIKE FLIES

It took forty years, but the free-radical theory of aging has now gained widespread support, earning Denham Harman a nomination for the 1995 Nobel Prize in Medicine. The reason for this increased acceptance is that there is now a significant amount of supporting data. Two corroborating experiments were conducted by Rajindar S. Sohal, Ph.D., a free-radical biologist from Southern Methodist University in Dallas. In his first experiment, published in 1985, Sohal raised male houseflies in two different living situations. He housed one group in cages large enough to allow the insects to fly. The second group was housed in containers too small to allow flight.

The flies that could fly, Sohal discovered, lived a maximum of 28 days, typical for a housefly, but the flies that could only crawl lived an amazing 65 days, more than twice as long.[5] Sohal attributed the longevity of the inactive flies to the fact that they consumed less oxygen, resulting in the generation of fewer oxygen-based free radicals. (Couch potatoes take note.) By lowering the incidence of free-radical damage, vital cells were preserved, resulting in the prolongation of life.

Sohal got similar results in 1994 using an entirely different approach. This time, instead of reducing the number of free radicals being generated, he found a way to mop them up after they had been created. In this high-tech experiment, he altered the genetic makeup of a group of fruit flies so they would have extra copies of the genes that produce the antioxidant enzymes catalase and superoxide dismutase. In a matter of weeks, the fruit flies with the extra helping of antioxidants were so energetic that Sohal could tell which group was which just by glancing at them. The antioxidant-supplemented insects also lived much longer—93 days, compared with 71 days for the normal flies. Sohal's experiment is regarded as the first definitive proof that bolstering the right antioxidant defenses can increase maximum life span.

Sohal's experiments left just one significant objection to Harman's free-radical theory of aging: Once organisms approach the end of their customary life span, the pace of aging accelerates. If free-radical damage is indeed fueling the aging process, then aging should proceed at a steady pace—unless, of course, organisms have a diminishing supply of antioxidants. But no one could show clear-cut evidence that antioxidants diminish as we age.

Our recent work at the University of Texas Health Science Center, coupled with the work of hundreds of my colleagues over the past four decades, may have supplied the missing piece to Harman's theory. There is a vital antioxidant that declines precipitously with age—melatonin. And melatonin is such a potent, versatile antioxidant that its gradual loss could explain why aging accelerates over time.[6] As the evidence of melatonin's antioxidant prowess mounts, more and more of my colleagues are suggesting that melatonin replacement therapy could result in a significant increase in the human life span.

WHAT CAN WE LEARN
FROM ANIMAL STUDIES?

A theory, however, is only a theory. Melatonin replacement therapy cannot be regarded as a viable anti-aging strategy until its ability to extend life has been demonstrated in living organisms. So far, melatonin has been studied in only a handful of animal longevity experiments, all but one conducted by Maestroni, and his colleagues, Conti and Pierpaoli.

The one independent study was published in 1995 by a group of Israeli scientists, spearheaded by my colleague Nava Zisapel, Ph.D. This study involved rats instead of mice. (This difference is significant because although rats and mice may appear similar, their genetic makeup is quite different.) The rats responded to melatonin just as dramatically as the mice. After fifteen months, 87 percent of the melatonin-treated rats were alive, compared with only 43 percent of those not given the hormone.[7] The experiment also provided new evidence of melatonin's ability to counteract the effects of aging on the immune system. In the control group, five of the seven surviving rats had severe pneumonia, while the melatonin-treated rats were completely healthy or had only very mild symptoms.[8] At the present time, a number of research groups around the country are making plans to replicate Maestroni's and Zisapel's studies.

EAT LESS—LIVE LONGER?

As we wait for the results from other melatonin studies, we can gather a few clues about melatonin from experiments involving other anti-aging strategies. The most effective and well-researched strategy is calorie restriction. If young animals are limited to 60 percent of their normal food intake, they live as much as 50 percent longer than animals given free access to food. In addition, the animals have a lower incidence of virtually all degenerative diseases and appear more youthful well into old age.

Researchers discovered the anti-aging effects of calorie restriction in 1934, but so far no one has been able to prove how or why it works, despite the millions of dollars that have gone into the effort. Now the mystery may be unraveling: The success of calorie restriction may rely to some degree on the body's ability to stimulate melatonin production. In 1991 my colleagues and I in San Antonio measured the melatonin levels of three groups of rats: (1) old rats that had been given free access to food, (2) old rats that had been raised on a low-calorie diet, and (3) young rats that had been freely fed. As expected, the old rats fed a normal diet had much lower melatonin levels than the young rats; an age-related decline in melatonin production has been seen in virtually all animals and humans studied to date. But the older underfed rats were producing *twice* as much melatonin as their well-fed peers. As you can see by the chart in Figure 28, they were also producing almost as much melatonin as rats one-fifth their age.[9] This suggests that calorie restriction and preserved melatonin production go hand in hand.

Further evidence linking calorie restriction with increased melatonin levels comes from a study published in 1978. The pineal glands were removed from aged rats that had been fed a low-calorie diet, then compared with the pineal glands of old rats fed a normal diet and with those of very young rats. The pineal glands of the food-deprived rats looked like the glands of the young animals, showing "a profound retardation of cell loss," compared with the freely fed animals.[10]

One implication that could be drawn from these studies is that the anti-aging effects of calorie restriction may depend to some degree on the preservation of a youthful supply of melatonin. There is one way to prove this contention: remove the pineal glands of rodents, *then* put them on a low-calorie diet. If they fail to exceed their

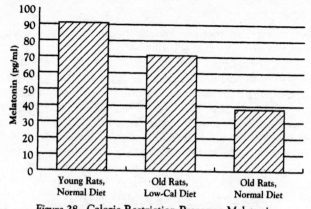

Figure 28. **Calorie Restriction Preserves Melatonin**
Older rodents that are fed a calorie-restricted diet have
melatonin levels of much younger animals.

normal life span, then melatonin is presumably essential
for the anti-aging effect.

GATHERING CLUES
FROM THE HEALTHY ELDERLY

What does human research suggest about melatonin's potential to extend our lifespan? Some indirect evidence can
be gleaned from studies of long-lived people. For instance,
if melatonin does indeed delay the aging process, then
individuals who exceed the average lifespan might have
relatively high levels of the hormone. A good population
to study in this regard would be women, because the fairer
sex has an enviable record for longevity. In the United
States, a baby girl born today has a 1-in-3 chance of living
to be 100. A baby boy has only a 1-in-10 chance of reaching the century mark. Gerontologists have been trying to
explain the "female longevity factor" for decades. In the
1960s, they hypothesized that women lived longer than

men because they led less stressful lives. In the 1970s, they suggested that women lived longer because fewer women than men smoked. In the 1980s, they concluded that women had the actuarial edge because estrogen protected their hearts. One by one, these theories have been shot down. All that gerontologists are willing to venture at this point is that the gender gap would still exist even if all environmental, behavioral, and social influences were eliminated.[11]

Is it possible that women live longer because they produce more melatonin? In order to answer this question, researchers would have to measure the melatonin levels of tens of thousands of people of all ages, which has yet to be done. At least four smaller studies, however, have awarded women the melatonin advantage. A French study conducted in 1985 compared the melatonin levels of 757 hospitalized male and female patients and discovered that the women produced an average of 25 percent more melatonin than the men.[12] A second study, this one a multinational study conducted by Swedish researcher Lennart Wetterberg and published in 1993, surveyed 321 healthy individuals and found that the women produced approximately 20 percent more melatonin than the men, even though, on average, the women had less body mass. A third study of 102 people revealed that women produced 30 percent more of the life-giving hormone than men.[13] Finally, a German study of 174 subjects detected higher levels of melatonin in older women compared with older men.[14]

If these findings are borne out in larger studies, it may be possible to conclude that the female longevity factor involves, among other things, an enhanced supply of melatonin.

HEALTHY ELDERLY VERSUS SENILE ELDERLY

Of all the ills that accompany aging, perhaps the most feared is loss of mental function. You can fight cancer and heart disease, but when you become senile, there is no "you" left to wage the good fight. Regrettably, senility is very common among the very old. One study suggests that almost half of all people over age 85 have Alzheimer's disease.[15] In the United States, an estimated 4 million adults have this form of dementia.[16]

But dementia is not the inevitable consequence of advanced years. Some people survive past the century mark with all their wits intact. What sets them apart? In 1993, Italian gerontologists studied the mental functioning of twenty-two elderly people and thirteen younger adults. They found a clear correlation between melatonin production and mental acuity. The better the patients performed on a test known as the Mini Mental State Exam, the higher their levels of melatonin.[17] A year later, a group of Japanese researchers produced a similar finding: The healthy elderly were producing more than twice as much melatonin as Alzheimer's patients of a similar age.[18]

Could a deficiency of melatonin contribute to the *cause* of Alzheimer's? Perhaps. Free radicals are believed to be a significant factor in the neuronal damage characteristic of Alzheimer's-type dementia. (One indication is that tissue taken from the brains of Alzheimer's patients at autopsy contain higher levels of a by-product of liquid peroxidation.)[19] Since melatonin may be the body's most potent antioxidant and is one of the few antioxidants to penetrate the blood-brain barrier, a person with a deficiency of this protective hormone is likely to suffer a greater amount of free-radical damage to the brain. Also, as we have shown at UTHSC, melatonin causes a significant increase in glutathione peroxidase, another antioxidant vital for the protection of the brain. Animal studies are now under way to see if melatonin supplementation can prevent some of the physical manifestations of Alzheimer's.

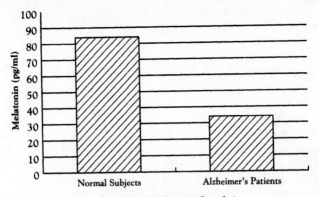

Figure 29. Low Melatonin Levels in
Alzheimer's Patients

In this study, Alzheimer's patients were producing much less
melatonin at night than people of a similar age who did not
show signs of dementia.

WHAT CAN WE LEARN FROM
THE OLDEST OLD?

Healthy people in their nineties and beyond are a rar-
efied group. Somehow they have managed to hold on
to a healthy cardiovascular system, fend off incipient
tumor cells, and triumph over a never-ending stream of
viruses and bacteria. Surely they have something to teach
us.

So far, no one has measured the melatonin levels
of these oldest old. But scientists from the University of
Parma in Italy have studied the immune responses of
twenty-three centenarians and come up with a finding
that may relate to melatonin: These individuals have a
highly aggressive population of natural killer cells, which
attack viral-infected and malignant cells. When their NK
cells were mixed in with cancer cells, they destroyed more
of the cancer cells than immune cells produced by people
forty or even fifty years younger.[20] Maintaining a healthy
population of NK cells could be one of the secrets of lon-

gevity. As we saw in Chapter 4, melatonin has a stimulatory effect on those very cells.

STIMULATING HUMAN GROWTH HORMONE

The anti-aging research community has a great deal of interest in human growth hormone, a product of the pituitary gland. When growth hormone is injected into aging humans, it stimulates muscle and bone growth, reduces body fat, enhances the immune system, and promotes a sense of overall well-being. In the future, when gerontologists concoct the ultimate anti-aging cocktail, growth hormone is likely to be one of its main ingredients.

But some people are not waiting for researchers to eke out data. They are flying to a health resort near Cancún, Mexico, and paying thousands of dollars for an initial screening and a three months' supply of the elixir. The potential benefits of growth hormone, they have decided, are worth the expense and inconvenience of a lifetime of frequent injections.

The relationship between melatonin and growth hormone is complex and not fully understood. Some studies have shown that melatonin has no effect on growth hormone, while others have shown it can either stimulate[21] or inhibit its production. The majority of the studies, however, suggest that melatonin has a stimulatory effect. In one of the most recent, eight adult men were given 10 milligrams of melatonin in the daytime and showed a slight increase in growth hormone levels. But when melatonin was given prior to administration of the hormone that stimulates growth hormone (growth hormone-releasing hormone, or GHRH), the result was a twofold increase in growth hormone.[22]

RESEARCH THAT NEEDS TO BE DONE

These studies offer tantalizing bits of evidence that melatonin may indeed prolong youth and vitality in humans. Clearly, more research is needed. One productive study would be to measure the melatonin levels of large numbers of older people to see how their pineal function relates to their health. In another experiment, supplemental melatonin could be given to older people to see if it caused any significant change in their immune response, blood pressure, cholesterol level, sleep patterns, or overall sense of well-being. If funding were available, these studies could be completed within a five-year time frame, allowing us to go into the twenty-first century with more insight into melatonin's anti-aging potential.

HOW MIGHT MELATONIN EXTEND HUMAN LIFE?

The possible mechanisms include:
1. **Reducing free-radical damage**
2. **Stimulating an aging immune system**
3. **Protecting the cardiovascular system**
4. **Stabilizing the body's biological rhythms**
5. **Restoring the nightly cycle of rest and repair**
6. **Stimulating the production of growth hormone**

In the meantime, some people have found the existing evidence compelling enough to begin a program of lifelong melatonin therapy. Many of these people, not surprisingly, are melatonin researchers like myself. We have seen such dramatic evidence of the hormone's anti-aging effects in animals and have been sufficiently reassured as to its safety that we have decided to experiment on ourselves.

Should *you* join us in the great anti-aging experiment? I cannot make that decision for you. My goal is to provide you with some basic information, point you in the direction of further research, and encourage you to discuss the information with your physician. Meanwhile, hundreds of researchers around the world are intently exploring melatonin's anti-aging properties. Stay tuned for further developments.

PART II

▼

ATTAINING HEALTHY LEVELS OF MELATONIN

CHAPTER 13

▼

LET THERE BE LIGHT—
AND DARK

In 1971, I began an unofficial experiment in my garage. I wanted to see if hamsters living without heat or air conditioning and with only sunlight for illumination would go through the same breeding cycles as the hamsters being housed at the medical school. Perhaps the conditions in our climate-controlled lab were too different from those in a natural setting, skewing our observations.

I situated the hamsters by the garage windows so they would be exposed to lots of daylight, but I blacked out the windows on the side facing the street so there would be no interference at night from the streetlights. By no means was a two-car garage in the suburbs of San Antonio a natural habitat for hamsters, but it was certainly less artificial than the animal room at the laboratory. At the laboratory, strict rules apply. For example, we have to keep the temperature at a constant 22 degrees centigrade (72 degrees F) night and day. The humidity must be maintained at 45 percent. Even though the animals in my garage weren't running free in the wild, they would at least be exposed to some sunlight and to seasonal changes in temperature and humidity.

At first I was interested only in the reproductive status of the two groups of hamsters, but as the months went by, my attention was drawn to another phenomenon—their health. For some reason, the hamsters in the garage seemed more fit than the ones at the lab. They were spunkier and had glossier coats. I remember saying to one of my colleagues, "The hamsters at home are happier than the ones here at work."

What was causing the difference? I couldn't be sure because there were far too many variables. It could have been the lighting, the temperature, the humidity, or a combination of all three. But if I had to place a bet, it would be on the lighting and its effect on melatonin.

A number of experiments I conducted in the following years helped confirm my suspicion, but the most applicable was one initiated in 1988 by a group in Finland. In their study, they kept one group of rats in a windowless room that was illuminated by fluorescent lights, and another group of rats in a room with natural sunlight. Unlike my ad hoc garage experiment, their experiment kept all the other factors the same, including temperature and humidity. The researchers even exposed both groups of animals to the same duration of light. When the sun rose, they switched on the lights in the windowless room; when the sun set, they turned them off.

After one week, the researchers measured the melatonin levels of the two groups and came up with a significant finding: The rats in the sunlit room were producing far more melatonin at night than the ones in the artificial lighting environment.[1]

What is it about sunlight that stimulated their nocturnal melatonin production? Sunlight differs from fluorescent light in a number of ways, including spectrum (the "color" of the light) and intensity. In the Finnish experiment, the most influential factor was the intensity. The intensity or brightness of light is measured in *lux*. The

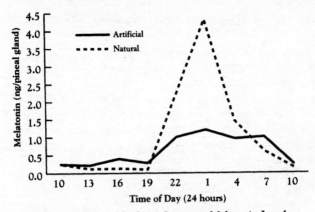

Figure 30. **Natural Lighting Increases Melatonin Levels**
Rats that were housed in a room with natural light produced
more melatonin at night than those exposed to artificial light.

light in the windowless room was kept at a constant 400 lux, which is brighter than the typical indoor environment. The light in the sunlit room varied from a few lux at dawn and dusk to as much as 3,000 lux on a bright sunny day—more than seven times the light of the fluorescent bulbs.

WHAT IS A LUX?

A lux is a measurement of light. To give you a frame of reference, 100 lux is the amount of light that would enter your eyes if you were looking at a 100-watt bulb from a distance of 5 feet in an otherwise dark room.

Another difference in lighting conditions was that in the windowless rooms the intensity of the light was ungraded; dawn came with a blast of fluorescent light, and night descended with the flick of a switch. During all the hours in between, the rats were exposed to a constant 400 lux. By contrast, the rats in the sunlit room experienced a smooth gradation of light from morning to night.

LIVING IN THE TWILIGHT ZONE

This study raises some important questions about the way our modern lighting environment might be influencing our own melatonin production. Like the rats in the windowless room, most of us spend very little time in the sun. For the most part, we work indoors. During our leisure time, we sit entranced in front of our television sets, video games, and home computers. Many of us exercise on treadmills rather than on sidewalks. We drive to the store and to church. We watch football rather than play it.

Just how little time we spend outside was revealed in a 1994 study conducted in sunny San Diego. On average, middle-class, middle-aged adults spent less than 4 percent of their time outdoors, and much of this time was spent in their cars.[2] People in less hospitable climates are likely to be even more house-bound. But the people who spend the most time in the dark are the nation's millions of night-shift workers: They are exposed to bright light for only 2.6 percent of their waking hours.[3]

How much light are we exposed to inside our offices, factories, and homes? Very little, according to Daniel Kripke, M.D., a researcher at the University of California at San Diego. He and his colleagues have measured the light exposure of more than a thousand people and found that a majority of those surveyed were exposed to light levels of less than 100 lux for much of the day.[4]

To put this finding into perspective, it helps to compare 100 lux with the range of light available outside. During the daytime it is rare for light levels to be less than 500 lux, even on a dark cloudy day. On a bright summer day the light outside can reach 100,000 lux. This is a thousand times more light than we are likely to experience indoors.

Figure 31 compares the amount of light that was available outdoors on a sunny April day in Seattle with the hour-by-hour light exposure of an office worker on the very same day. The office worker's greatest light exposure occurred while driving to and from work, which is true for many of us urban dwellers.

DOES BRIGHT LIGHT INFLUENCE YOUR PRODUCTION OF MELATONIN?

Whether bright light increases nighttime production of melatonin in humans is still being debated, but at least four studies have shown that it does. Barbara Parry, M.D., associate professor at the University of California at San Diego, has focused much of her attention on women with premenstrual syndrome (PMS), one of the many conditions that has been linked with low melatonin levels. When women with PMS are exposed to two hours of bright artificial light during the day, she found, they produce more melatonin at night.

Three Australian researchers found an increase in mel-

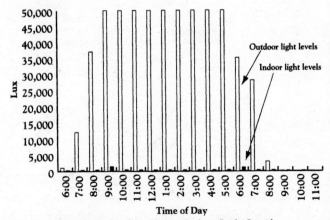

Figure 31. **Outdoor Versus Indoor Light Levels**

This chart shows the amount of light available outside on a sunny day compared with the light exposure of an office worker on the very same day. The indoor lighting levels are barely visible on this scale.

atonin levels when they administered light therapy to SAD patients. According to their 1990 report in *Lancet*, "almost all [nocturnal melatonin] concentrations were higher after successful treatment than they had been at equivalent times before phototherapy."[5] In a similar study conducted in Germany, thirty patients with nonseasonal depression underwent one week of light therapy. Prior to the therapy, only 21 percent of the depressed patients had a significant rhythm of melatonin. After the therapy, this figure increased to 47 percent.[6] The graph in Figure 32 shows the dramatic increase in melatonin levels in one of the participants.

In yet another study, light therapy raised the melatonin levels of people suffering from insomnia. Before light exposure, the insomniacs had considerably lower levels of the hormone than people without sleeping difficulties. For five consecutive mornings, the insomniacs spent half an hour in front of a light box. At the end of the study, they were producing 160 percent more melatonin at peak times during the night.[7]

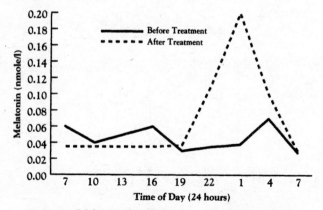

Figure 32. **Melatonin Levels Increase After Light Therapy**
Light therapy increased nocturnal melatonin production in a patient.

HOW DOES BRIGHT LIGHT
AFFECT YOUR MIND AND YOUR MOOD?

In 1993 fifteen men and women in their twenties and thirties spent four hours in bright light (2,500 lux) and then four hours the next day in moderate light (500 lux). Before being exposed to the light, and then periodically throughout each period of light exposure, various tests measured their physical and mental condition. In a test of their reaction time, they made fewer errors after being exposed to bright light than to the dimmer light. (Plant managers take note.) Significant improvements after bright light were also found in their cognitive function, wakefulness, and reaction time. Most important, under the bright-light conditions, the volunteers reported a much greater sense of well-being.[8]

What accounts for these remarkable changes? One possibility is increased levels of serotonin, melatonin's parent molecule. Serotonin is the neurotransmitter that is enhanced by antidepressant drugs such as Prozac, Zoloft, and Paxil. In a 1992 study, researchers measured the serotonin levels of two groups of volunteers before and after light therapy. One of the groups was composed of people with depression and the other group were healthy controls. Following light therapy, both groups showed a significant increase in serotonin, but the depressed group benefited even more than the nondepressed group.[9]

Natural sunlight may have a similar antidepressant effect. Dr. Rachele Espiritu, one of the San Diego light researchers, discovered that people who spend a considerable amount of time outside have few depressive symptoms, especially the symptoms associated with SAD—overeating, social avoidance, and fatigue.[10]

HIGH SEROTONIN IN THE DAY,
HIGH MELATONIN AT NIGHT—
A RECIPE FOR HEALTH

A high level of serotonin during the day punctuated by a strong pulse of melatonin at night appears to be nature's formula for vibrant good health. Serotonin keeps you alert and energized during the daytime; melatonin helps you rest and recuperate at night. I believe it is significant that both of these vital substances may be enhanced by exposure to bright light during the daytime. Our primitive ancestors were farmers or hunter-gatherers, spending much of their time out of doors. Our lifestyle has changed drastically since those times, but our bodies very little. In our ignorance, we have estranged ourselves from the sun, creating yet another health hazard—light deprivation.

We would do well to heed some ancient teachings. The *Tao Tsang,* a two-thousand-year-old Chinese text, teaches that "exposing the eyes to direct sunlight greatly benefits the brain by stimulating secretions of vital essences there."[11] We happen to call those vital essences melatonin and serotonin, but my guess is that the Chinese sages were describing the same phenomena. The yogic tradition maintains that the pineal gland is the "crown chakra" through which solar radiation energizes the body.[12] The Bible proclaims, "The lamp of the body is the eye. If your eyes are sound, you will have light for your whole body, if the eyes are bad, your whole body will be in darkness" (Matthew 6:22–23).

With their lux meters and light boxes and intricate study designs, medical researchers have buttressed these beliefs with scientific data. No matter which tradition one follows—an Eastern spiritual tradition, the Christian tradition, or the scientific tradition—the message is the same: For optimum physical and mental health, we need to crawl out of our urban caves and spend more time in the light.

DEPRIVED OF DARKNESS

When night comes, however, it's just as important that we retreat from the light and embrace the healing power of darkness. Dark conditions allow our pineal glands to produce melatonin, triggering a much-needed time of rest and repair. Unfortunately, to the same degree that we are light-deprived during the daytime, we are darkness-deprived at night. When the sun sets, we turn on the lights, shrinking the night to the seven or eight hours we spend sleeping. Illuminating the nighttime may make our lives more pleasurable and productive, but we pay a hidden price: We deprive ourselves of a significant portion of our natural supply of melatonin.

Twenty-five years ago, melatonin researchers believed that light suppressed melatonin production in animals but not in humans. We humans were too intelligent or highly evolved to behave in such a primitive fashion, they thought. The person who disabused them of this notion is Alfred Lewy, a leader in the field of light therapy and melatonin research. In a landmark paper published in 1980, Lewy demonstrated that light of sufficient brightness (2,500 lux) can cause a significant reduction in nighttime production of melatonin.[13] Since then, it's been shown that far less light—as little as 100 lux—can inhibit the nighttime production of melatonin in some people. Many of us are exposed to light of this intensity at night on a regular basis. The brighter the light, the greater the dip in one's melatonin production.

As in most things, however, people vary a great deal in their response to light. In one study, 500 lux of light suppressed melatonin production by 8 percent in one person but an amazing 98 percent in another.[14] There is some indication that people with low levels of melatonin are most vulnerable to the suppressive effect of light.[15] In other words, the less melatonin you have, the more you stand to lose. Another group of people who may be especially sensitive to light exposure are those who take extra vitamin B-12 (more than the recommended daily requirement). High amounts of this particular vitamin can cause melatonin production to drop more dramatically in response to light at night and take longer to recover once the light is turned off.[16] A new and intriguing piece of research suggests that women as a group may respond to light more strongly than men. In a study published in 1995 in the *Journal of Neural Transmission*, six women and six men were exposed to bright light in the middle of the night. In dark conditions, there was no significant difference in their melatonin levels. Once bright lights were turned on, however, the women had a forty percent greater reduction in melatonin levels than the men, indicating that women may be more vulnerable to the negative effects of light at night.

How long must you be exposed to bright light at night before your melatonin production is inhibited? As little as five minutes, according to a 1989 study.[17] To my knowledge no one has studied the effects of a shorter exposure. In some laboratory rats, a one-second pulse of light is enough to lower their melatonin levels, but it is generally agreed that people are far less sensitive.

SLEEP DEPRIVATION MAY DEPLETE YOUR SUPPLY OF MELATONIN

The fact that bright light suppresses melatonin production has serious implications for the millions of adults in this country who are chronically sleep-deprived—they may be melatonin-deprived as well. By itself, being awake does not shut down melatonin production. If you were to lie wide awake at night in a dark room, you would produce just as much melatonin as if you were sound asleep. But, most people who habitually shortchange themselves on sleep tend to spend their waking hours in lighted environments. If the light is sufficiently bright, they may be robbing themselves of a potent anti-aging, cancer-fighting, free-radical-scavenging hormone.

The amount of time we spend sleeping has declined steadily within this century until we are now sleeping 20 percent less than did people in the early 1900s. As a result, an estimated 30 million adults and teenagers in the United States are chronically sleep-deprived. According to a 1992 report, people who sleep six or fewer hours a night are in poorer health and have a 70 percent higher mortality rate than those who sleep a full seven or eight hours.[18]

They may also have a diminished immune response. Recently, twenty-three healthy men volunteered to be awakened at three in the morning (after four hours of sleep) and then stay awake for the rest of the night. Following this truncated sleep, the researchers measured the men's immune responses and then compared them with a night when the men had gotten a full eight hours of sleep. Shortchanging the men on sleep, they found, caused an average 28 percent reduction in natural killer cell activity.[19] Given the fact that melatonin *stimulates* natural killer cells, this reduction could be caused by a lack of melatonin.

HOW TO PRESERVE YOUR
NATURAL SUPPLY OF MELATONIN

To retain your full allotment of melatonin, you may have to make some changes in your lifestyle. You may, for one thing, have to increase your exposure to light in the daytime. How much daylight exposure is necessary for optimum health and well-being? Some studies suggest you should spend at least an hour a day in light levels that exceed 1,000 lux. This amount of light is not available indoors unless you sit in front of a specially designed light box or look out a window on a sunny day. It is estimated that only 5 percent of adults get this minimum amount of light exposure.[20]

Spending more time out of doors is an ideal way to increase your light exposure. Taking a "light break" during the day or eating lunch outdoors could make a great deal of difference. Another solution is to get most of your exercise outdoors. People who participate in outdoor sports such as golf, tennis, swimming, hiking, biking, jogging, fitness walking, camping, or boating are likely to have a much greater exposure to sunlight than those who exercise in a home or gym.

Unfortunately, being outside also increases your exposure to UV light, which is a known risk factor for skin cancer and eye disease. Dermatologists recommend that you wear sunscreen whenever you are outside—rain or shine. (Blocking UV light from penetrating your skin will *not* reduce your melatonin production; the only light that increases melatonin is believed to be the light that comes through your eyes.) On a bright day, however, you should also protect your eyes. The trick is to purchase a pair of sunglasses that offer UV protection but are lightly tinted so that an adequate amount of light can enter your eyes.

You can take some simple measures to increase the level of light inside your home or workplace as well. Open your drapes and blinds during the day. Locate your favorite chair or desk next to a window. Trim away shrubs and bushes that block the light from entering your house. Paint your walls with a light-colored paint. All these measures may greatly increase your daily light intake. Installing three-way bulbs or dimmer switches in your home will allow you to bask in bright light during the daylight hours but have subdued lighting at night.

If you are building or renovating your home, consider bringing in more natural light by adding greenhouse windows, skylights, or "sun tubes," tubes that channel light into your house. If you have a yard, you might want to add a sheltered area where you can sit outside during the day and still be protected from the wind, rain, and direct rays of the sun.

Other small changes in your daily routine can further increase your light exposure. For example, while waiting at the airport, choose a seat that faces the windows. Make a habit of sitting in a window seat on a plane, bus, or train. Bring in an extra lamp to brighten your space at work. If you have a sun roof on your car, drive with it open as much as possible. Pull down the sun visor only when necessary to block the direct rays of the sun.

DECREASING LIGHT AT NIGHT

For your health and well-being, it is just as important to minimize your light exposure at night, particularly in the hour or two before bedtime, when your nocturnal melatonin production is on the rise. If you read at night, turn on just enough light to be able to read comfortably. Turn the lights down or off while you watch TV. If too much light comes in through your bedroom windows, add darker shades or curtains. If your partner is reading in bed while you want to sleep, wear a sleep mask. If you wake up at night to go to the bathroom, keep the lights low. (A night light in the hallway or bathroom may be sufficient to light your way.)

Get more sleep. According to Dr. James Maas, a professor of psychology at Cornell University, 90 percent of us need eight hours or more a night.[21] Some people are very sensitive to their need for sleep and can tell immediately if they are sleep-deprived; other people are less aware of their sleep needs. Three tests will tell you if you are among the millions of sleep-deprived individuals. (1) Turn off your alarm clock and see if you still wake up in the morning at your regular time. If not, you are probably short-changing yourself on sleep. Ideally, you should go to bed early enough so that you wake up (fully rested) before the alarm rings. (2) Lie down in the middle of the afternoon in a darkened quiet room. If you fall asleep in fewer than five minutes, you may not be getting enough sleep at night. (3) If you nod off at work or school or have difficulty staying awake while driving, you may be *seriously* sleep-deprived.

By setting aside more time for sleeping, you will reward yourself with a longer cycle of nocturnal melatonin production. Being suffused with melatonin will lower your blood pressure, stimulate your immune system, and allow you to cycle through all the normal stages of sleep. You will awaken the next day with a rejuvenated mind and body.

CHAPTER 14

▼

THE ELUSIVE ENEMY— ELECTROMAGNETIC FIELDS

About twenty years ago, two Denver researchers, Nancy Wertheimer, Ph.D., and Ed Leeper, Ph.D., began to search for a link between childhood leukemia and environmental hazards. The incidence of leukemia among children was increasing significantly, suggesting to Wertheimer that some change in the environment might be responsible. She scrutinized the records of hundreds of leukemia patients but found no clear-cut link with any known environmental hazard. She did, however, discover a potential new one—extremely low frequency electromagnetic fields, or EMFs,[1] an invisible form of energy that is created whenever electricity flows through a wire. Among children living in homes located near electrical transformers (the large canisters attached to power poles), she found, the mortality rate was two to three times higher than among children living in homes without this exposure.

Prior to Wertheimer's discovery, EMFs were thought to be a harmless form of radiation. One reason EMFs were believed to be safe is that they vibrate or oscillate at a leisurely 50 or 60 times a second, which is referred to as 50 or 60 hertz. By comparison, your favorite FM radio station is beamed to you on waves that oscillate 100 *million* times per second, or 100 megahertz (MHz). X-rays oscillate at 1,000,000,000,000,000,000 times a second (1 quintillion, or 10^{18}). The higher the frequency, the more energy is contained in the fields and the more damage they seem to cause. Gamma radiation, at the top end of the radiation scale, has enough energy to rip electrons from molecules, potentially causing a tremendous amount of cell damage.

HOW DO SOURCES OF ELECTROMAGNETIC FIELDS RANK IN TERMS OF FREQUENCY?

In descending order of hertz:

Gamma rays	10^{20}
X-rays	10^{18}
Ultraviolet	10^{16}
Visible light	10^{15}
Infrared	10^{12}
Microwaves	10^{10}
Radio waves	10^{6}
EMFs	10^{1}

Note: To convert these numbers from scientific notation into everyday numbers, add as many zeros as the number in the superscript. For example, the hertz of visible light, which is 10^{15} Hz, is the same as 1 followed by 15 zeros, or 1,000,000,000,000,000 Hz.

The Denver leukemia study prompted some scientists to question the safety of EMFs. The concern grew in following years as statistical links were found between EMFs and other kinds of cancer, including melanoma, lymphoma, brain cancer, prostate cancer, and breast cancer. More recently, other conditions have been added to the list, most notably spontaneous abortion, depression, and Alzheimer's disease.

MELATONIN—THE SMOKING GUN?

But what do EMFs have to do with melatonin? For many years, scientists were unable to pinpoint any mechanism by which EMFs could cause cancer and other diseases. Although a number of possible explanations were offered, none emerged as definitive. Now, there is the growing suspicion that EMFs could contribute to some or all of these diseases by interfering with the action of melatonin. In three different situations—the use of electric blankets in the home, exposure to EMFs in a laboratory setting, and exposure to a medical imaging device called an NMR (nuclear magnetic resonance spectroscopy)—EMFs have lowered melatonin levels in some people.[2] Some scientists have gone so far as to call the EMF-melatonin connection the "smoking gun" that assures a guilty verdict for EMFs. This connection, however, is far from proven.

CLOCK, CALENDAR, AND COMPASS

We had no idea that EMFs had any effect on melatonin until the early 1980s, when a German zoologist named Peter Semm began investigating animal migration. One of the ways migrating birds orient themselves, Semm knew, is by detecting subtle changes in the earth's energy fields, the magnetism that emanates from electrical currents deep within the earth. (These fields are the reason that a compass points north.) Semm wanted to know how animals detect these invisible energy fields. He reasoned that migrating animals need to orient themselves in both time and space to rendezvous at their chosen destinations. It was known that seasonal changes in melatonin production sent a time cue that caused "migratory restlessness," compelling animals to band together and strike out for distant lands.[3] He theorized that the pineal gland might also serve as a direction finder. After all, the gland is highly responsive to light, which is a *visible* form of electromagnetic energy. Perhaps it tuned in to lower frequency fields as well, Semm thought.

He tested his hypothesis on guinea pigs, applying magnetic fields to the heads of the rodents. The fields reduced the electrical activity of individual pineal cells by as much as 50 percent, he found. His intuition had been correct. A year later, a group of American researchers led by Bary Wilson exposed rats to electric fields for twenty-one days and discovered that the fields abolished their nighttime rise in melatonin production.[5] Other studies have shown that magnetic fields (as opposed to electric fields) may also influence the ability of the pineal gland to produce melatonin at night.

These discoveries may have uncovered yet another function of the multitalented pineal gland. We now believe the gland links organisms with time and space in three vital ways: It synchronizes them with the twenty-four-hour day, it triggers seasonal changes, and it may also detect fluctuations in geomagnetic fields. In essence, the gland seems to function as a clock, calendar, and compass, answering these three vital questions—"What time of day is it?" "What is the season?" and "Where am I on the planet?"

▶ CROSSED WIRES

Unfortunately, the all-purpose pineal gland has one major failing: It does not discriminate very well between natural and man-made energy fields. When migratory birds are placed in cages surrounded by electrical coils, these artificial energy fields conflict with the earth's geomagnetic fields, sending confusing messages to the animals. No longer able to obtain a true compass reading, the birds may head off for Anchorage instead of Cancún. Similarly, pigeons that have been outfitted with portable magnets find it much harder to wend their way home. Whales also rely on geomagnetic fields to help chart their migrations; it may be interference from man-made energy fields that causes some of them to beach themselves in shallow lagoons.

▶ THE HUMAN COMPASS

Such cross-wiring may take place in our own human brains. The first experimental evidence that the human pineal gland responds to natural energy fields came in 1986. Rolf Dubbels, Ph.D., a friend and colleague of mine from Germany, was making routine measurements of melatonin levels in a small group of men wintering in Antarctica. At one point, an outburst of solar flares (sunspots) caused the local magnetic field to plummet. During the most intense night of the magnetic storm, three out of seven men had a threefold change in their melatonin levels, suggesting that we humans may also be vulnerable to fluctuations in the geomagnetic field.[6]

Aeons ago, when humans were primarily hunters and

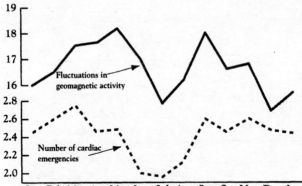

Figure 33. **Monthly Average of Daily Cardiac Emergency Cases**
There is a striking correlation between the amount of geomagnetic activity in a given month and the number of people admitted to hospitals with heart problems.

gatherers, we, too, may have relied on our pineal glands to orient ourselves in space. Whether we rely on our compass today is not known, but it may produce some inadvertent effects. Biometeorologists, who study the effects of the weather and meteorological events such as geomagnetic fields on living organisms, have found a number of statistical links between sudden changes in the earth's magnetic fields and human health and behavior. Births and deaths, epileptic seizures, homicides, admissions to mental hospitals, and heart attacks—the rates of all have been correlated with fluctuations in geomagnetic activity. A study published in *Nature* in 1979 revealed that geomagnetic activity (for example, intense solar storms) is correlated with the number of people suffering heart attacks.[7] As you can see in Figure 33, the correlation is striking.

A study published in *The British Journal of Psychiatry* in 1994 reports that two weeks after an intense geomagnetic storm, as many as 36 percent more male manic depressives may be admitted to mental hospitals, which the authors suggested could be due to complex interactions between the pineal gland and magnetic fields.[8]

DO ARTIFICIAL ENERGY FIELDS AFFECT PRODUCTION OF MELATONIN?

As disconcerting as it may be that our pineal glands respond to geomagnetic fields, it may prove far more significant that they respond to *man-made* energy fields. Although the evidence is preliminary, magnetic fields from ordinary household wiring and appliances may lower melatonin levels in humans. In a study yet to be published, researchers measured the EMF exposure of forty California women as they went about their daily routines. Some of the women happened to be electric-blanket users. When they slept with their blankets turned on, their melatonin levels were as much as 50 percent lower than when they did not use the blankets.[9] While the women were snug and warm under their electric blankets with their heads nestled close to their EMF-generating alarm clocks, the EMFs were sending errant messages to their pineal glands, robbing their bodies of one of their most influential hormones.

But the link between EMFs and the human pineal gland is far from clear. Other studies have shown that EMFs do *not* have an inhibitory effect on melatonin production. This contradiction is not surprising, given the difficulties involved in measuring melatonin levels, our lack of knowledge of which parameter of the energy fields to measure, and the great diversity among the human population. It may be years, if not decades, before we have any definitive answers.

EMFs, MELATONIN, AND BREAST CANCER

If EMFs *do indeed* cause a significant reduction in melatonin levels in humans, the implications are many. One possibility is an increased risk of cancer, especially breast cancer. Richard Stevens, Ph.D., a researcher at Battelle Northwest, an independent research agency in Washington, was the first person to theorize a link between EMFs, melatonin, and breast cancer. For many years he had been curious about the dramatic rise in the incidence of breast cancer in the United States. In 1940 an American woman who lived to age 85 had a 1-in-20 chance of having breast cancer; today that risk has risen to 1 in 8.

Like many other people, Stevens conjectured that our urban lifestyle might be making women more vulnerable to breast cancer. But what specific aspect of that lifestyle was to blame? Some researchers had implicated diet, stress levels, and exposure to toxins. EMFs had also been considered, but no one had found the mechanism by which they might promote cancer. Stevens did some investigating and turned up the fact that EMFs may lower melatonin levels in animals. Could this be a possible mechanism? His curiosity piqued, he learned all he could about melatonin. Eventually he found the clue he was looking for: Melatonin had been shown to reduce the risk of breast cancer in animals. Now Stevens had the basis for a theory linking EMFs with breast cancer: (1) Melatonin may help protect against breast cancer; (2) EMFs have the potential to lower melatonin levels; and (3) EMFs may promote breast cancer *indirectly* by lowering melatonin levels. Although this theory was strung together with qualifying words like *potential*, *may*, and *could*, it had its merits. Stevens published his theory in 1987, one year after David Blask announced that melatonin slows the growth of breast cancer cells. These two papers prompted researchers to begin searching for statistical data to prove or disprove the theory.

▶ THE STATISTICAL LINK BETWEEN EMFs AND BREAST CANCER

Supportive data has in fact been found. Researchers in Seattle found a sixfold increase in breast cancer among male telephone linemen, electricians, and electrical power workers. Norwegian scientists found a fourfold increase in the risk of breast cancer in male electrical transport workers. Researchers at the University of North Carolina found a 40 percent higher mortality rate from breast cancer in female electrical workers.[10]

More data comes from an animal study published in 1995. Rats that were injected with a cancer-causing chemical (DMBA) and then exposed to electromagnetic fields had markedly larger tumors than those injected with DMBA alone.[11] The researchers concluded that their findings "add to the accumulating evidence that MF [magnetic field] exposure exerts tumour co-promoting effects."[12] Stevens's theory linking EMFs with breast cancer is now buttressed with both statistical and experimental evidence.

▶ **EMFs BLOCK THE ANTICANCER ACTIVITY OF MELATONIN**

The potential causal link between EMFs, melatonin, and breast cancer has been further strengthened by a test-tube study conducted by Robert Liburdy, Ph.D., a researcher from the University of California at Berkeley. Liburdy discovered that magnetic fields interfere with melatonin's ability to slow the growth of breast cancer cells, a new and potentially important insight. Other researchers had found that EMFs may lower the amount of melatonin in the bloodstream; Liburdy found that EMFs may block melatonin's *actions*. This implies that even if you have adequate amounts of melatonin—or take melatonin supplements—EMFs may render the hormone impotent, depriving you of its anticancer action.

Liburdy gained this insight by culturing human cancer cells in a melatonin solution. (As David Blask had shown, melatonin should cause a significant reduction in the growth of the cells.) He then exposed the cells to a moderate level of magnetic fields, 12 milligauss. (This is about the same exposure you would get standing in front of an electric range with a front burner on high.) After seven days, he measured the rate of growth of the cells and found that they had grown just as quickly as cells that had *not* been cultured with melatonin. Magnetic fields—those invisible, omnipresent fields that bathe us from morning to night—*had blocked melatonin's cancer-fighting ability*.

THE POLICY OF PRUDENT AVOIDANCE

The research showing that EMFs may be harmful to your health is in its earliest stages. Much of the data gathered so far is either incomplete or contradictory, and it may be years or even decades before we understand why. Given the lack of definitive data, people are lining up on both sides of the issue. Alarmists would have us believe that

EMFs are decimating our society. At the other end of the spectrum are those who have labeled the entire issue "the electromagnetic hoax."[13]

What's the truth of the matter? I wish I had the definitive answer. For the past few years I have served on two committees to evaluate the scientific literature as to the possible biological effects of EMF exposure. (One of these panels was convened by Dr. Allan Bromley, the scientific adviser to then-President George Bush. The other committee was sponsored by the National Academy of Science.) The consensus of both of these groups is that while EMFs may cause biological changes in living organisms, there is no conclusive evidence at this time that they cause negative health effects. In the meantime, the National Institutes of Health is sponsoring a $65 million, four-year research program to gain additional insight. Results of this research should be available in the late 1990s.

In the meantime, what should you do? For several years, many experts on electromagnetic fields have been recommending a policy of "prudent avoidance." Prudent avoidance means taking simple inexpensive steps to reduce your exposure to EMFs. If man-made energy fields turn out to be harmless, you will not have wasted a great deal of time and money. But if they turn out to be hazardous, you will have benefited from your timely actions.

If you want to reduce your exposure to EMFs, you need to know how to pinpoint EMF "hot spots." EMFs are not present in uniform fields throughout your home and workplace. Rather, they come from discrete sources, most typically from household wiring, electrical appliances, and outdoor power lines. The strength of these fields falls off dramatically with distance. The farther away you are from an EMF-generating source, in other words, the lower your exposure. For example, if you are standing right next to a dishwasher, you may be exposed to as much as 800 milligauss. If you step back just one foot, your exposure drops to 12 milligauss. Another two feet, and the level drops to a barely measurable amount.

What is a safe level of EMFs? We don't know. Somewhat arbitrarily, scientists have decided that 2 milligauss and below is a "low" or "safe" level of exposure, but there is no guarantee that even this low amount is free from negative effects.[14]

One reason we don't know if exposure to 2 milligauss is safe is that we have no data from a control population—that is, from a large group of people with no exposure to artificial electromagnetic fields. All the data we have comes from studies comparing people exposed to a high amount of EMFs, like electrical workers, with those who are exposed to average fields. This is like comparing the health of two-pack-a-day smokers with one-pack-a-day smokers. It tells us nothing about the risks of very low levels of EMFs versus no exposure. Some of the health problems we now regard as commonplace could be due to the low level of electromagnetic fields present in a typical home or work environment.

▶ HOW TO DETERMINE YOUR
   EMF EXPOSURE AT HOME

EMF levels vary greatly from household to household. Depending on the location of your home, the kind of wiring in your walls, and the number and placement of electrical devices, you may be living in a high-, moderate-, or low-risk environment. The only way to know with any certainty is to measure the fields directly. To do so, you can hire an electrical consultant, take advantage of free services that may be offered by your utility company, or measure them yourself with a special instrument called a gaussmeter (*Gauss* rhymes with *house*). These devices are also referred to as EMF detectors.

Buying your own gaussmeter has some advantages. Having one at your disposal means you can survey your home and workplace as thoroughly as you like and then monitor any changes that occur over time. You can also take measurements at night, which is when your pineal gland may be most vulnerable. And you can monitor electrical appliances *before* you buy them. Electromagnetic fields produced by similar electrical devices vary in strength to a surprising degree. For instance, one brand of electric shaver emits 14 milligauss at a distance of four inches, while another sends out a staggering *1,600* milligauss.

A high-quality EMF detector can cost three hundred dollars or more. Less costly ones are available, but they won't give you a precise reading in milligauss. Instead, they emit a beeping sound when they detect EMFs above a certain level. This may be all the information you need. (See the Resources section for more information.)

You can also learn a great deal about your EMF exposure by studying the Strength of Electromagnetic Fields chart that follows. It shows you at a glance the wide range of electromagnetic fields emitted by similar products, and the dramatic decrease in your exposure with distance.

STRENGTH OF ELECTROMAGNETIC FIELDS
(in Milligauss)

APPLIANCE OR TOOL	DISTANCE FROM SOURCE		
	4 inches	1 foot	3 feet
Fan	20–900	75–200	5–20
Can opener	130–4,000	30–300	.5–7
Electric shaver	14–1,600	1–90	.1–3
Vacuum cleaner	230–1,300	20–200	1–20
Electric massager	150–420	20–75	.5–1.5
Hair dryer	13–300	1–6	—*
Microwave oven	200–600	40–90	3–5
Electric pencil sharpener	120–800	15–70	.5–1
Power saw	200	40	5
Electric drill	150	30	5
Cordless drill	20	<1	—
Television	5–100	.4–20	.1–1.5
Portable heater	100–200	5–20	1–2
Electric range	30–90	10–18	1–3
Copy machine	90	20	7

Fluorescent light	12–40	2–6	—
Computer monitor (VDT)	14–600	3–30	1–2
Computer	1–4	< 1	—
Baby monitor	6	1	—

— indicates a negligible amount.

Some of the worst offenders are devices with electrical motors, such as electric drills, can openers, pencil sharpeners, vacuum cleaners, electric massagers, and table saws. Virtually all major kitchen appliances are in the high range. Microwave ovens produce two kinds of energy fields: microwaves and EMFs. The microwaves are confined within the oven by special shielding devices, but the EMFs radiate into the room. Fluorescent lights contain an electrical device called a ballast that produces EMFs. If the lights are several feet above your head, they are not likely to be much of a hazard. Fluorescent desk lamps, on the other hand, may be close enough to your body to expose you to excessive levels of EMFs.

Computer monitors (but not computers themselves) generate significant amounts of electromagnetic fields, especially out the sides and back of the case. Newer models tend to emit lower levels than older ones. When shopping for a new monitor, look for ones that meet or exceed Swedish MPR II Standards. You can purchase filters that reduce the glare and/or electrical fields of computer monitors, but they do *not* block magnetic fields. The devices that lower both electric and magnetic fields are considerably more expensive and may need to be specially ordered. There are several companies that will retrofit your old monitor with internal shields.

Television sets also emit EMFs, but they are less of a potential hazard than computer monitors because you tend to sit farther away from them. Surprisingly, black-and-white televisions produce more EMFs than color sets. When your mother told you to "scoot back from the TV," she was right.

KEEP YOUR DISTANCE

A person who wants to minimize exposure to EMFs would do well to follow this simple rule—Keep your distance. If you stay at least an arm's length away from an appliance, your exposure is likely to be very low. Unfortunately, some sources of EMFs are not visible, such as the wiring inside walls. You may not know exactly where the wiring is located, nor what kind of wiring it is. In general, wiring that has been installed within the past few decades emits fewer EMFs than wiring found in older buildings. You may need to hire an electrician or EMF consultant to determine your actual exposure.

One simple precaution you can take right now is to locate where the main power supply comes into your house or apartment. All of the electricity you use is funneled through this one spot, resulting in high levels of EMFs. To minimize your exposure, do not place furniture that gets frequent use (beds, easy chairs) in this area.

MONITORING SPECIFIC AREAS OF YOUR HOME

You spend as much as a third of your life sleeping, so reducing your EMF exposure in the bedroom may be especially important. Place all electrical devices, including clocks, telephone answering machines, electrical transformers, radios, and stereos two feet or more from your bed. Analog alarm clocks (the kind with clock face and hands) generate a lot of EMFs; keep them at least three feet away. In the nursery, make sure that all electrical devices (including baby monitors) are three or more feet from the crib.

Electric blankets are in a special category for five separate reasons: (1) they expose your entire body to EMFs; (2) they are in close contact with your body; (3) they have been reported to lower melatonin levels in some people; (4) they have been associated with a slightly higher risk of miscarriage and cancer; and (5) you use them at night, when your pineal gland is actively producing melatonin.[15] To minimize your exposure, you have a number of options. The first, of course, is to refrain from using an electric blanket. The second is to use one to warm your bed and then turn it off before you retire. The third and least recommended is to use an electric blanket throughout the night but select one that is specifically designed to reduce EMF exposure. (Check the label or call the manufacturer for details.)

Electrically heated waterbeds pose some of the same problems. To eliminate the risk, turn off the heating element before you get into bed. In cool weather, preserve the heat throughout the night by using a specially designed insulating pad.

Your entire kitchen may be an EMF Hot Zone. As you cook dinner, you may be encircled by half a dozen electrical devices, including a portable TV, electric range, dishwasher, refrigerator, microwave oven, toaster oven, and food processor. When several of these appliances are turned on, every area in your kitchen may have EMF levels above 2 milligauss.

You can reduce your exposure, however, by making some simple changes. The heating element in your dishwasher may produce high levels of EMFs. By letting your dishes air dry or by drying them by hand, you can reduce some of this exposure. Or simply run your dishwasher when you are out of the room. When you are cooking, stand back as far as possible from the electric range or microwave oven. If possible, relocate the microwave oven so that it is out of the way. If you have an electric range, consider converting to a gas appliance.

In the bathroom, hair dryers and electric shavers expose you to high levels of EMFs because you hold them close to your head. Consider switching to a plain razor or a battery-operated shaver, and forgoing the hair dryer or holding it as far as possible from the head. (A 1991 survey found the highest correlation between childhood leukemia and the use of two specific electrical appliances—hair dryers and black and white TV sets.[16]) Battery-operated appliances, such as cordless drills, toothbrushes, and shavers, are considered safe.

In time, monitoring your exposure to EMFs will become second nature. You will become more mindful of electromagnetic fields when you make decisions about where to live, where to send your children to school, how to arrange your furniture, which appliances to buy, where to locate them, and how to use them. The key words to remember are "prudent avoidance"—a comfortable middle ground between being unduly alarmed and ignoring the possible danger.

CHAPTER 15

▼

DRUGS THAT DEPLETE MELATONIN

Of all the known ways to diminish your body's supply of melatonin, perhaps the simplest and most effective is to take a standard dose of certain well-known prescription or over-the-counter medications. The list of drugs that deplete melatonin includes such common products as aspirin, ibuprofen, beta-blockers, calcium channel blockers, sleeping pills, tranquilizers, and at least one well-known antidepressant. So-called recreational drugs—caffeine, tobacco, and alcohol—can also be found on the list. The chances are very good that you or someone you love is unwittingly taking a substance that is sabotaging the production of melatonin.

What are the long-term consequences of taking melatonin-lowering drugs? Theoretically, it could increase your free-radical damage, make you more vulnerable to cancer, depress your immune system, increase your risk of degenerative disease, and even shorten your life span. But since no one has conducted a long-term study to test this hypothesis, we can only speculate.

A great deal of clinical evidence is available, however, about the *short-term* effects of most melatonin-lowering drugs, and at least some of these effects may be due to their inhibitory effect on melatonin. In the pages that follow, I will look at each of these drug classes in turn and suggest ways that you can lower their negative impact on your melatonin production while retaining their benefits.

NSAIDS

Nonsteroidal anti-inflammatory drugs, or NSAIDs (pronounced "en-seds"), are a family of pain relievers that includes aspirin, ibuprofen and indomethacin. Volunteers who took just one normal dose of aspirin or ibuprofen in the evening had as much as a 75 percent reduction in melatonin levels.[1] This reduction is greater than you would get from sleeping under an old-fashioned electric blanket or staying awake all night in a brightly lit room. "Take two aspirin and call me in the morning" may no longer be sage medical advice.[2]

Of all the NSAIDs, indomethacin may cause the greatest reduction in melatonin levels. In one study, a slow-release preparation of indomethacin was given to volunteers at six in the evening. The pain-killer caused a "complete blockade of the nocturnal increase" of melatonin.[3] In other words, the volunteers produced no more melatonin at night than they did during the day.[4]

NSAIDs also cause sleep problems, perhaps because they rob the body of its best nighttime sleep aid. In a 1994 double-blind study, researchers at Bowling Green State University studied the effects of aspirin, ibuprofen, and acetaminophen (a non-NSAID drug) on sleep. The volunteers slept in the lab overnight while the researchers monitored their sleep with various recording devices. The results showed that aspirin and ibuprofen interfered with

sleep, but acetaminophen did not. The researchers speculated that the fact that the NSAIDs "suppress the nocturnal surge in melatonin synthesis . . . may have played a
role in altering sleep patterns."[5]

NSAIDs can also increase blood pressure and interfere with antihypertensive drugs such as beta-blockers.[6]
This negative side effect may also be caused by their inhibitory effect on melatonin production. (As we saw in
Chapter 7, melatonin has the potential to reduce blood
pressure.)

What pain-reliever should you take at night if you want
to prevent these negative effects on your melatonin production? All of the common pain-relievers tested so far
have had a negative effect on the hormone. The fact that
acetaminophen caused the least sleep problems in the
Bowling Green study suggests that it may have a lesser
effect on melatonin production, but preliminary data suggests that it, too, may lower melatonin levels.[7] If your pain
is mild enough that it does not disturb your sleep, you
might be wise to take your last pain-reliever before dinner.
Consult your physician for advice.

Many arthritis sufferers rely on these drugs extensively
to cope with their pain. What options do they have? Dr.
Billie Sahley at the Pain and Stress Center in San Antonio recommends melatonin itself to arthritis sufferers. "So
far we've seen excellent results. They are reporting a remarkable decrease in pain."

Another possibility is to take aspirin or another pain-
reliever at night but then supplement it with melatonin.
A young woman with severe menstrual cramps reported
that her doctor prescribed high doses of NSAIDs for her
during the first part of her menstrual cycle. The NSAIDs
relieved her pain, but disrupted her sleep and gave her
nightmares. But if she took 3 milligrams of melatonin
along with the NSAIDs, she found, she got both pain
relief and a good night's sleep. Ask your doctor for advice.

People who are taking aspirin to reduce their risk of
heart attack and stroke might do well to take the tablets
in the morning. Although they will still have aspirin in

their bloodstream at night (aspirin has a very long half-life), the amount will be diminished.

HEART MEDICATIONS

▶ BETA-BLOCKERS

Beta-blockers are a type of drug prescribed for a variety of heart problems, including high blood pressure, abnormal heart rhythms, and angina. They include such products as propranolol (Inderal), atenolol (Tenormin), and metoprolol (Lopressor, Toprol). Beta-blockers get their name from their ability to block or interfere with "beta-adrenergic receptors," key cell receptors. When these receptors are blocked, your heart pumps less forcefully and your arteries relax, lowering your blood pressure and easing angina. But beta-receptors are found on other key organs, including the pineal gland. When you take a beta-blocker to lower your blood pressure, the drug may disrupt your production of melatonin as well.

Pineal researchers knew decades ago that beta-blockers abolish melatonin production in lab animals. During our research, it is sometimes necessary to deprive animals of their melatonin supply, to see how they function without it. One way to do this, as we have seen, is to remove their pineal glands. Another and more humane way to achieve the same end is to give them a beta-blocking drug such as propranolol. Beta-blockers are so effective at stopping melatonin from being synthesized that we refer to their use as a "pharmacological [drug-induced] pinealectomy."

In 1992, G. M. Braun, M.D., demonstrated that beta-blockers are equally effective at stopping human melatonin production. In the graph in Figure 34, the top line shows the melatonin level of a person before taking a beta-blocker. The flat line below shows the melatonin level of the same person after taking a low dose of propranolol. (The dose was 50 milligrams. Typically, patients take at least 80 milligrams of propranolol a day, with a maximum recommended dosage of 640 milligrams.)[8]

As with NSAIDs, beta-blockers have a number of negative side effects that could be explained by their inhibitory effect on melatonin production. For example, many people who take beta-blockers suffer from insomnia, restless sleep, strange dreams—even nightmares. (This is also true for people who take ophthalmic beta-blockers such as timolol for glaucoma. Even though these drugs are given as eye drops, they can enter the circulatory system and affect the entire body.)

In 1988 a group of Swedish researchers explored the possible relationship between the sleep-disturbing effects of beta-blockers and their known ability to block melatonin production. The researchers tested three different kinds of beta-blockers—propranolol, atenolol, and metoprolol. They found that volunteers who were given metoprolol had the steepest decline in melatonin levels and the severest sleep problems. "In the metoprolol group," the researchers noted, "a significant relationship was found between the fall in melatonin and the percentage of disturbed nights. Severe CNS (central nervous system) side effects, such as nightmares, occurred only in

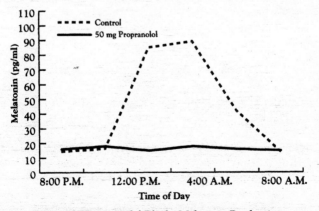

Figure 34. Propranolol Blocks Melatonin Production

patients treated with metoprolol, which in all cases were accompanied by low levels of melatonin. Our data suggests that the CNS side effects during beta-blockade are related to a reduction of melatonin levels."[9]

Another possible side effect of metoprolol is to raise cholesterol levels.[10] This unwanted action could also be caused by the drug's melatonin-lowering property, because melatonin has been shown to inhibit cholesterol production.[11] To my knowledge, no one has investigated this connection.

▶ CALCIUM ANTAGONISTS OR CALCIUM CHANNEL BLOCKERS

This new generation of heart medications includes bepridil (Vascor); diltiazem (Cardizem); felodipine (Plendil); isradipine (DynaCirc); nicardipine (Cardene); nifedipine (Adalat, Procardia); nimodipine (Nimotop); and verapamil (Calan, Isoptin).[12] Calcium antagonists work by blocking special channels that allow calcium to enter the various cells in the cardiovascular system. This action causes the arteries to relax and decreases oxygen demand by the heart.

Unfortunately, calcium channel blockers may not discriminate between the cells in the heart and the cells in the pineal gland. When you take one of these drugs, calcium could also be restricted from entering your pineal cells. But calcium is vital for melatonin production. In fact, the two areas of the brain with the highest concentrations of water-soluble calcium are the pineal and pituitary glands.

A 1986 animal study examined the effects of calcium channel blockers on melatonin production. Four different kinds of calcium channel blockers were given to a group of young baboons. Three of the four medications— nisoldipine, nifedipine, and nitrendipine—caused significant reductions in nocturnal levels of melatonin. The greatest suppression occurred when the drugs were given at night. The fourth medication, verapamil, had no apparent effect on melatonin production.[13]

Taking a calcium channel blocker early in the day may minimize its inhibitory effect on the production of melatonin and may give you other benefits as well. A 1994 article in *Hypertension* reported that taking nitrendipine before breakfast lowers the customary early morning surge in blood pressure. This surge is associated with an increased risk of heart attack and stroke. Also, the average blood pressure of the subjects was lowest when the drug was taken before (not after) breakfast.[14]

Yet another high blood pressure medication that reduces melatonin is clonidine. Clonidine (Catapres) is referred to as an alpha-receptor blocker. When clonidine is administered at night, it causes a significant reduction in melatonin levels. The greater the dosage, the greater the suppressive effect.[15]

► MINIMIZING THE NEGATIVE EFFECTS OF
  ANTIHYPERTENSIVE MEDICATIONS

If you are now taking a blood pressure medication that lowers your melatonin levels, should you stop taking it? Absolutely not. The drug may be essential for your health. (I take mine faithfully.) You may, however, be able to reduce the melatonin-lowering effects of these drugs. Ask your doctor if you can take your hypertensive medication first thing in the morning. By nighttime, the level of the drug in your blood will have declined, minimizing its possible effect on your melatonin production. If you must take the drug in the evening, discuss with your doctor the possibility of taking supplemental melatonin as well.

You could consider switching to an alternative form of treatment. There are a number of techniques for lowering blood pressure that do not rely on antihypertensive medications. Weight loss, exercise, reduced salt consumption, and lowered alcohol intake are some of them. Certain vitamins and minerals (calcium, magnesium, and vitamin

B-6) have also been shown to have an antihypertensive effect. Finally, with your doctor's approval, you may try taking melatonin itself. As we saw in Chapter 7, it appears to cause a significant reduction in blood pressure in some people. A doctor who emphasizes nutrition and preventive care is likely to be most knowledgeable about these alternatives.

ANTI-ANXIETY DRUGS AND SLEEP AIDS

At least two widely prescribed anti-anxiety drugs, diazepam (Valium) and alprazolam (Xanax[16]), inhibit melatonin production.[17] Both of these medications belong to a family of drugs called benzodiazepines (which were discussed in more detail in Chapter 8). In one study, volunteers who took 2-milligram doses of Xanax at nine P.M. had reduced melatonin levels throughout the night.[18]

Both alprazolam and diazepam are prescribed with some frequency for short-term relief of insomnia. But the sleep they produce is different from normal sleep. Alprazolam, for example, may alter the amount of time you spend in priority sleep.[19] Melatonin, which does not change normal sleep pattern and has anti-anxiety properties as well, may prove to be a superior sleep aid.

ANTIDEPRESSANTS

Many antidepressant drugs stimulate melatonin production. Examples include fluvoxamine (Luvox)[20], desipramine (Norpramin, Pertofrane), and most MAO inhibitors (Marplan, Nardil, Parnate, and others.) But the most popular antidepressant drug, fluoxetine (Prozac), which has annual sales in the United States of more than a billion dollars, could *lower* your melatonin levels. A study published in *The British Journal of Psychiatry* in 1995 reports that depressed patients who took fluoxetine had significantly lower nocturnal melatonin levels after one week of use. Subjects who were not depressed who took fluoxetine also had lower melatonin levels after one week, and their levels declined even further after six weeks of use.[21]

Like most antidepressant drugs now on the market, Prozac has a number of negative side effects, some of which could be caused by adverse effects on melatonin production. Insomnia, which affects a significant number of Prozac users, is a likely candidate.[22] There is no data to support this contention, but given the fact that melatonin enhances sleep, research into this possible connection seems warranted.

VITAMIN B-12

Some people take large doses of Vitamin B-12 (methylcobalamine or cyanocobalamin) in an effort to relieve stress, increase their energy level, or cure pernicious anemia. But this practice may also deplete their melatonin supply. In a 1992 Japanese study, nine healthy men were given three daily doses of vitamin B-12 for a total of 3 milligrams a day. Compared with the placebo, vitamin B-12 caused a significant decrease in their average twenty-four-hour melatonin levels.[23] (Vitamin B-12 is contained in most multivitamin preparations, but usually in such small doses that it is unlikely to influence melatonin production.)

CAFFEINE

Coffee has been used for centuries to increase alertness, but we learned only recently that it achieves this end, in part, by blocking the production of melatonin. Given caffeine's reputation for disturbing sleep, it's remarkable that no one explored the caffeine-melatonin connection until

1994. Dr. Kenneth Wright, Jr., and his colleagues at Bowling Green State University measured the melatonin levels of a group of individuals who volunteered to stay awake for two consecutive days. Some were given a placebo and others were given 200 milligrams of caffeine, which is equivalent to two cups of strong coffee. (Eight ounces of instant coffee contains approximately 65 milligrams of caffeine. Freshly brewed coffee ranges from 75 to 120 milligrams.) Compared with the placebo, caffeine caused a significant reduction in their melatonin levels.[24]

Volunteers who took caffeine and were also exposed to bright light had a further reduction in melatonin levels. Not surprisingly, they did better on performance tests and found it easier to stay awake than those who took caffeine alone or were treated only with bright lights.[25] Next time you are struggling to stay awake on the job or to study for an exam, you can use this information to good advantage: Turn up the lights and pour on the java. On the other hand, if you want to *sleep* at night, turn down the lights and, as is well known, stay away from caffeine. One study determined that drinking coffee at eight o'clock at night

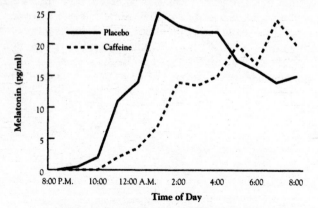

Figure 35. Caffeine Lowers Melatonin Levels
Volunteers given caffeine tablets equivalent to two cups of coffee had a significant drop in melatonin levels for the next eight hours.

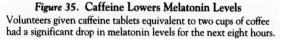

lowered melatonin levels for at least six hours.[26] (The half-life of caffeine is between six and nine hours.)

Many people claim that they can drink coffee at night and still sleep soundly. But studies have shown that most of these people sleep less soundly and wake up more often than they are aware.

While coffee contains the most caffeine, other beverages contain goodly amounts of the stimulant as well. Black tea, for example, has approximately 40 milligrams per eight ounces. (Green tea has 25 milligrams of caffeine; most herbal teas have none.) Many soda drinks contain caffeine as well. At the top of the list is Jolt Cola with a hefty 71.2 milligrams per twelve ounces, but other sodas are not far behind. Drinking two cans of some of the following beverages is equivalent to drinking one cup of strong coffee.

Brand of Soda	Caffeine (milligrams per 12 ounces)[27]
Jolt	71
Mountain Dew	52
Tab	44
Sunkist Orange	42
Dr Pepper	38
Diet Dr Pepper	37
Pepsi-Cola	37
Diet-Rite	34
Diet Pepsi	34
Coca-Cola	34
7-Up	0
Sprite	0
Diet 7-Up	0
Fresca	0
Hires Root Beer	0
Diet Sunkist Orange	0

I regret to say that chocolate also contains a significant amount of caffeine, especially dark chocolate, which is more concentrated than milk chocolate. Having a piece of dark chocolate cake and a cup of coffee at the end of a meal is an invitation to insomnia.

KIND OF CHOCOLATE	CAFFEINE (milligrams)
Dark chocolate (1.5 ounces)	31
Semisweet chocolate chips (1/4 cup)	33
Milk chocolate (1.5 ounces)	9
Hot chocolate (5 ounces)	8

Caffeine can cause a number of negative side effects in addition to insomnia, including anxiety, cardiac arrhythmia, and upset stomach. Pregnant women who drink caffeine with regularity have an increased risk of having low-birth-weight infants. Caffeine may also increase the risk of spontaneous abortion, raise cholesterol levels, increase blood pressure, and increase the risk of atherosclerotic heart disease. In fact, a 1992 study of 9,484 men found a small but significant association between coffee consumption and all causes of death.[28] Whether caffeine's suppressive effect on melatonin contributes to any of these negative side effects is open for speculation. (Some pain-relievers, such as Excedrin, contain both NSAIDs and caffeine. This combination of ingredients taken at night or in the late afternoon is likely to cause an even greater reduction in your melatonin levels.)

STEROIDS

The steroid drug dexamethasone is prescribed for a variety of conditions, including asthma, lymphoma, shock, lupus, bursitis, tendinitis, and arthritis. It is known to cause serious sleep disturbances in patients, including insomnia and vivid, frightening, or morbid dreams. Dexamethasone also reduces melatonin levels. A study published in *The Journal of Pineal Research* in 1988 found that one milligram caused a significant reduction in melatonin levels in nine of eleven volunteers. Their peak levels declined from an average of 127 to 73 picograms per milliliter.[29] (Dexamethasone is prescribed in doses ranging from 0.5 to 16 milligrams.)

TOBACCO

At least two studies have suggested that people who smoke cigarettes have lower nighttime melatonin levels than people who don't.[30] One of the studies, published in 1994, reported that "all the smokers had lower melatonin levels than non-smokers. The relation between smoking and melatonin concentrations needs to be further studied."[31]

Smoking tobacco has some very serious and well-publicized side effects, including a greatly increased risk of heart disease, cancer, respiratory disease, and peptic ulcers. A forty-year study of male British doctors concluded, "It now seems that about half of all regular cigarette smokers will eventually be killed by their habit."[32]

A lesser side effect of smoking is insomnia. A survey of 3,516 adults showed a relationship between smoking and fragmented sleep. Smokers had more difficulty falling asleep and found it harder to get up in the morning. Female smokers complained of excessive daytime sleepiness, while men reported nightmares and disturbing dreams.

Could the sleep problems and more serious difficulties associated with smoking be related to low melatonin levels? We don't know. But if smokers need yet another reason to curb the habit, tobacco's potential to interfere with melatonin production can now be added to the list.

ALCOHOL

A 1993 study showed that volunteers who drank the equivalent of one or two glasses of wine at seven o'clock in the evening had 41 percent less melatonin at midnight compared with nights when they were given a nonalcoholic drink. When they were given higher doses of alcohol, they had low melatonin levels until the early hours of the morning.[33]

Could this be why alcohol disrupts sleep? Although alcohol may ease anxiety and help you fall asleep, it can produce a rebound effect several hours later, leaving you wide awake and staring at the clock. Studies have shown that alcohol decreases both REM sleep (dreaming) and delta sleep, which is the most restorative part of the sleep cycle. It also increases the number and duration of awakenings throughout the night.[34]

Paradoxically, alcohol may *stimulate* melatonin production when it is consumed very late at night. In a study published in 1995, alcohol was given to eighteen volunteers at eleven P.M. Fifteen of the eighteen subjects had significantly *higher* levels of melatonin for the next three hours.[35] Perhaps a late-night drink is a viable way to *increase* your melatonin production. (An acquaintance of mine says that her healthy and active ninety-two-year-old grandmother swears by her nightly dose of peppermint schnapps.) I suggest you wait for further studies, however, before you resort to this method. Drinking alcohol on an empty stomach may increase your risk of ulcers.

SUBSTANCES THAT MAY DECREASE MELATONIN

Acetaminophen	Bepridil
Alcohol	Caffeine (coffee, tea, and some soda drinks)
Alprazolam	
Aspirin	Clonidine
Atenolol	Dexamethasone
Benzerazide	Diazepam

Diltiazem
Filodipine
Flunitrazepam
Fluoxetine
Ibuprofen
Indomethacin
Interleuken-2
Isradapine
Luzindole
Methylcobalamine
Metoprolol
Nicardipine

Nicotine
Nifedipine
Nimodipine
Nisoldipine
Nitrendipine
Prazosin
Propranolol
Reserpine
Ridazolol
Tobacco
Vitamin B-12

CHAPTER 16

▼

CREATING A MELATONIN-FRIENDLY LIFESTYLE

Thy food shall be thy medicine.

—Hippocrates (460–377 B.C.)

A truly good physician first finds out the cause of the illness, and having found that, he first tries to cure it by food. Only when food fails does he prescribe medication.

—Sun Ssu-Mo, Tang Dynasty (A.D. 600)

Normal resistance to disease *never* comes out of pill boxes. Adequate food is the cradle of normal resistance, the playground of normal immunity, the workshop of good health, and the laboratory of long life.

—Charles Mayo, founder of the Mayo Clinic (1915)

What you eat you are.

—George Harrison, "Savoy Truffle," 1968

In the summer of 1993, I was in Lauenbruck, Germany visiting my friend and colleague Rolf Dubbels. Dubbels is an avid gardener. As he was giving me a tour of his well-tended vegetable garden, he turned to me and asked, "Do you think there is any melatonin in vegetables?" I said, "Well, people have found melatonin in algae and a few plants, so I wouldn't be surprised." He decided to investigate. Using a complicated technique, he searched for melatonin in nine common foods, including cucumbers, bananas, and tomatoes. He found melatonin in all of the plants he tested, the amount varying considerably from one kind to another.[1]

Dubbels's discovery prompted a postdoctoral student in my lab, Atsuhiko Hattori, Ph.D., to launch a similar investigation. In short order, Hattori determined the melatonin levels of twenty-four additional edible plants. Then he went one step further and fed a group of lab animals food that was especially rich in melatonin. The melatonin was absorbed into the animals' bloodstream, giving them significantly higher levels of the hormone in their serum, an effect that lasted for hours.[2]

This plant research could have direct influence on your health and well-being. If you want to raise your melatonin levels naturally, you might start by eating a bedtime snack of foods high in melatonin. This simple practice may help you sleep better, strengthen your immune system, heighten your antioxidant protection, and partially offset the age-related decline of melatonin production.

Which foods are rich in melatonin? The research has just begun. For now, the richest source of melatonin appears to be a grass plant called tall fescue. Those who drink grass juice—yes, there are people who swear by it—can add a new item to their juicing menu.

For those of you who are reluctant to graze your way to better health, please refer to the following list, which ranks food items in order of melatonin content.

FOODS HIGH IN MELATONIN

Food	Melatonin (picograms per gram)
Oats	1,796
Sweet corn	1,366
Rice	1,006
Ginger	583
Tomatoes ("Sweet 100s")	500
Bananas	460
Barley	378

Connoisseurs of Japanese food can add these foods to their list:

Japanese radish	657
Ashitaba	623
Chungiku	417

The list is short, but with a little imagination you can concoct a number of bedtime snacks from these ingredients. For starters, try a banana. When you tire of plain bananas, try a banana-milk "smoothie." (Mix a banana and 1/2 cup milk in a blender or food processor.) Experiment with the grains. Munch on toasted oatmeal, cooked oatmeal and bananas, oat granola, rice, rice cakes, rice pudding, rice cereal, rice noodles, corn bread, corn muffins, or corn flakes. For variety, fix yourself a bowl of tomato soup. As you try these various foods, note which ones make you the sleepiest. It may be a good indication of how much melatonin is getting into your bloodstream.

When should you eat these foods? If you are trying to influence your sleep, eat them an hour or so before bedtime. During this time your melatonin level can rise, easing you into sleep. Otherwise, eat your snack shortly before lights out, so the effect will last as long as possible throughout the night.

Is it mere coincidence that most of the foods on this list are known to have special healing properties? Bananas, for example, reportedly promote sleep, lower cholesterol, help prevent and heal stomach ulcers, and keep DNA from being damaged (antimutagenic). Oats lower cholesterol and blood pressure. Tomatoes are antimutagenic and inhibit the growth of certain tumors. Rice bran is claimed to be a potent antioxidant. Ginger soothes the stomach, eases menstrual cramps, stimulates the immune system, reduces cholesterol, and shrinks liver tumors in animals. Is melatonin responsible for some of these health-giving effects? We have yet to explore the possible connection.

TRYPTOPHAN INCREASES MELATONIN PRODUCTION

If this were the 1980s, I would suggest another way to raise your melatonin levels—take tryptophan tablets. Tryptophan is an essential amino acid, one of the building blocks of protein that we cannot synthesize within our bodies and therefore must get from our diet. Tryptophan is the molecule from which melatonin is derived. Your pineal gland synthesizes melatonin by converting tryptophan to serotonin and then to melatonin. Studies have shown that if you increase your intake of tryptophan, you increase your production of melatonin.[3] Figure 36 shows the effects of taking one gram of tryptophan at bedtime.

Unfortunately, tryptophan is no longer available in most countries because a small number of contaminated lots were sold in the late 1980s.[4] More than fifteen hundred people contracted a disease called eosinophilia-myalgia syndrome (EMS). One-third of them were hospitalized, and twenty-four died.[5] Although we now believe that tryptophan itself was not to blame, the sale of the amino acid is still banned. The resolution of this matter may one day make tryptophan available again.

Even though you cannot purchase tryptophan itself, you can increase the level of the amino acid in your bloodstream by eating foods rich in tryptophan. As you may have heard, turkey and milk are relatively high in

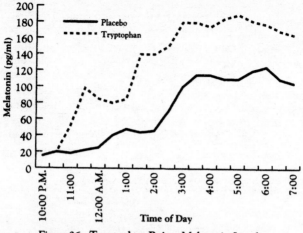

Figure 36. Tryptophan Raises Melatonin Levels
Taking one gram of tryptophan at night causes a
significant rise in melatonin levels.

tryptophan, but they are not the most abundant sources.
Numerous foods on this list contain even more of the
amino acid.

Foods Rich in Tryptophan	
Food	Tryptophan (mg.)
Spirulina seaweed (dried, 2 oz.)	580
Soy nuts (1/2 cup)	495
Cottage cheese (1 cup)	346
Chicken liver (3 1/2 oz.)	332
Pumpkin seeds (1/2 cup)	328
Instant breakfast (with 1 cup milk)	325
Turkey (3 1/2 oz.)	323
Chicken (3 1/2 oz.)	320
Tofu (1/2 cup)	310
Watermelon seeds (dried, 1/2 cup)	222
Almonds (1/2 cup)	204

Peanuts (1/2 cup)	176
Brewer's yeast (1 oz.)	150
Malted milk (1 cup)	125
Milk (1 cup)	113
Ice cream (1 cup)	100
Yogurt (1 cup)	67

VITAMINS AND MINERALS

Taking certain vitamins and minerals along with your bed-time snack may further enhance the production of melatonin. Niacinamide (nicotinamide, or vitamin B-3) is one of them. Your body has the capacity to make niacinamide out of tryptophan. If you supply the niacinamide ready-made, you free up some of the amino acid that could be used for conversion to melatonin. (Niacinamide by itself is recommended for insomnia and high blood pressure.) Natural sources of niacinamide include dried apricots, barley, beef liver, brewer's yeast, chicken, halibut, peanuts, pork, salmon, sunflower seeds, swordfish, tuna, turkey, veal, and wheat bran.

Another B vitamin, vitamin B-6 or pyridoxine, may stimulate melatonin production because the body uses it to convert tryptophan into serotonin, the precursor for melatonin. Animals can be deficient in melatonin even when they are only moderately deficient in vitamin B-6.[6]

If this is true for humans as well, then many people need to increase their vitamin B-6 intake. A majority of Americans have an inadequate intake of this B vitamin, especially the elderly, who are most in need of melatonin. More than 80 percent of the healthy, independently living, middle-income elderly surveyed in Albuquerque had intakes below three-fourths of the recommended daily allowance.[7] Less affluent elderly, the researchers speculated, might have even lower levels of B-6. Other people at high risk for a vitamin B-6 deficiency are smokers, drinkers, women who take birth control pills or estrogen, people with carpal tunnel syndrome, those who eat large amounts of refined foods, and people suffering from depression. The combined total of all these groups represents a majority of people in this country.

The similarities between the effects of vitamin B-6 supplementation and melatonin supplementation are striking. Both substances have been shown to lower blood pressure, lower cholesterol, relieve pain, relieve depression, stimulate the immune system, and reduce some of the behavior problems associated with autism and hyperactivity. To what degree the beneficial effects of B-6 are related to its ability to stimulate melatonin production is not known.

Foods high in vitamin B-6 include avocados, bananas, brewer's yeast, carrots, filberts, lentils, liver, rice, salmon, shrimp, soybeans, sunflower seeds, tuna, wheat bran, wheat germ, and whole wheat flour. Many enriched breakfast cereals are also relatively high in vitamin B-6. The fact that bananas contain a goodly amount of vitamin B-6 is yet another reason to choose this particular fruit as your bedtime snack.

CALCIUM AND MAGNESIUM

Today, as milk falls out of favor and carbonated beverages surge in popularity, a growing number of people are becoming calcium deficient. Calcium and magnesium are both vital to the production of melatonin. In fact, one study has shown that animals fed a calcium-deficient diet had shrunken pineal glands. Taking calcium and magnesium in the evening hours may have the greatest impact on your nocturnal melatonin production. According to one researcher, "A high calcium content at lights out may be necessary for the processes leading to the nocturnal increase in melatonin production."[8]

It is not known precisely which amounts of the vitamins and minerals I've mentioned produce optimum levels of melatonin, although a study that is now under way may provide the answer. But for the present you might start with 100 milligrams of niacinamide, 25 to 50 milligrams of vitamin B-6, 1,000 milligrams of calcium, and 500 milligrams of magnesium.[9] Ask your physician if there is any reason you should not be taking these supplements in these amounts. What time of day should you take these supplements? Take the niacinamide, calcium, and magnesium just before going to bed. However, the B-6 should be taken early in the day because it may make you feel more alert and energized, interfering with your sleep.

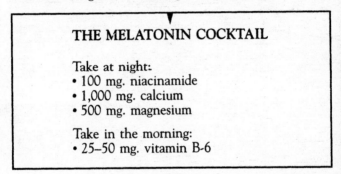

THE MELATONIN COCKTAIL

Take at night:
• 100 mg. niacinamide
• 1,000 mg. calcium
• 500 mg. magnesium

Take in the morning:
• 25–50 mg. vitamin B-6

MEDITATION

Reducing stress could be an effective way to increase your melatonin production. Researchers at the University of Massachusetts Medical Center measured the nighttime melatonin production of eight women who meditated regularly and compared them with the nighttime levels of eight nonmeditating women. The meditating women had significantly higher amounts of the hormone. This is yet another instance where your state of mind may be influencing your state of health. The researchers suggested that the pineal gland is "psychosensitive"[10]—350 years after

René Descartes wrote that the pineal gland is the "confluence of soma and psyche," or body and soul.

MARIJUANA

Of all the known ways to stimulate melatonin production, none is more dramatic than smoking marijuana. Marijuana stimulates production of a prostaglandin called PGE_2, which may relate to its ability to stimulate melatonin production. Italian researchers discovered that when eight men smoked a cigarette containing the active ingredient in marijuana, THC (tetrahydrocannabinol), they had dramatically higher melatonin levels twenty minutes later. After two hours, their melatonin levels were 4,000 percent higher than at baseline![11]

The fact that smoking marijuana is accompanied by a dramatic increase in melatonin production may explain some of the drug's positive effects. A 1995 article in *The Journal of the American Medical Association* reported that the hallucinogen is being used to counteract the toxicity of chemotherapy, treat migraines, reduce intraocular pres-

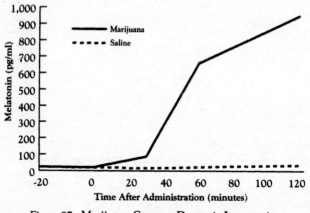

Figure 37. Marijuana Causes a Dramatic Increase in Melatonin Levels

sure, minimize pain, treat menstrual cramps, and moderate wasting syndrome in AIDS patients.[12] Melatonin has been shown to ameliorate each and every one of these conditions.

Smoking marijuana as a vehicle to increase melatonin production, however, is not a good idea. The increase is so marked that it is not likely to be beneficial, especially if one smokes marijuana during the daytime, when melatonin levels are normally so low that they are just above the level of detection. Causing such a dramatic surge in melatonin levels in the daytime could phase-shift your circadian rhythms or interfere with your health in other as yet unknown ways.

MAKING LIFESTYLE CHANGES

Throughout the book, I've discussed a number of ways to protect and enhance your natural production of melatonin. Some of these suggestions are simple to follow, such as decreasing your exposure to light at night or switching from one type of medication to another. But others may require you to change some ingrained behaviors, which could be quite difficult. For example, it may not be easy to change your sleep habits or to cut down on your consumption of tobacco or alcohol. If you are motivated to make some changes but find it difficult to do, I encourage you to get help.

A number of clinics, programs, and support groups around the country specialize in helping people make healthy changes. Your local hospital, for example, may have courses on meditation, stress reduction, yoga, and improving sleep habits. You may also benefit from working with a clinic or physician who is aware of the importance of maintaining a melatonin-friendly lifestyle.

RECOMMENDATIONS FOR A MELATONIN-FRIENDLY LIFESTYLE

- Increase your daytime exposure to sunlight or bright artificial light—ideally, first thing in the morning.

- Sleep long enough at night that you wake up feeling fully rested.

- Avoid bright lights at night.

- If possible, avoid night-shift work and travel that involves frequent crossing of time zones.

- Reduce your exposure to electromagnetic fields.

- Do not smoke. Drink in moderation.

- If possible, avoid melatonin-lowering drugs, or take steps to minimize their impact on your melatonin production.

- Eat foods rich in calcium, magnesium, vitamin B-6, and niacinamide, or take supplements of these vitamins and minerals.

- Eat foods rich in antioxidants or take antioxidant supplements.

- Eat snacks high in tryptophan or melatonin last thing at night.

- Spend some time each day in restful contemplation, meditation, or prayer.

CHAPTER 17

▼

TAKING MELATONIN
SUPPLEMENTS

In addition to taking steps to preserve and enhance their natural production of melatonin, many people take melatonin supplements. There are a number of reasons why this may be beneficial. If you are 60 or older, for example, creating a melatonin-friendly lifestyle may not be sufficient to restore your youthful supply of the hormone. Even if you are careful to get enough sleep, avoid light at night, and take a walk outdoors every day, you may still not produce enough melatonin. As you age, the machinery involved in the production of melatonin wears down. The SCN loses vital neurons; the lenses of the eyes become more opaque, blocking the entry of light; the pineal gland has fewer active cells, and fewer receptors on those cells. The net effect is a diminished supply of melatonin. People 70 and older may produce less melatonin at night than young people do in the daytime.

Second, many people have diseases or conditions that respond best to pharmacological doses of melatonin.

Those with moderate to severe insomnia, for example, may find they sleep somewhat better if they limit the use of melatonin-lowering drugs and eat a melatonin-enhancing snack before going to bed, but they may need even higher levels of the hormone to experience the best quality sleep.

Finally, some people may find it difficult to make all the lifestyle changes that are necessary to preserve their melatonin rhythm. I'm a case in point. I *know* I should be getting eight hours of sleep every night, but I rarely do. I travel too frequently and have too many demands on my time. Therefore, I am limiting the amount of time I allow my body to rest and repair. But even if I were to get a full night's rest every night, I would *still* take melatonin at night because I have reached the age where my melatonin-making machinery is beginning to wear down. I don't want to deprive myself of my best antioxidant so every night, I take a 1-milligram tablet before going to bed. My wife takes melatonin as well, both to help her sleep and to enhance her antioxidant protection.

The question I want to help you answer in this chapter is whether *you* should take melatonin. This question deserves careful consideration. Melatonin has great promise, but many of its uses have been so recently discovered that we have little information about dosage and protocol. We don't know, for example, how much melatonin to take for maximum anti-aging effects or for the greatest protective effect on the cardiovascular system.

Given this lack of knowledge, some researchers in the field are concerned about the number of people now taking melatonin. One of them is Cliff Singer, M.D., a sleep researcher at the Oregon Health Sciences University in Portland. Singer urges patience. "Melatonin research *is* being funded. The pace is slow and steady, but that is how the edifice is built, step-by-step, brick-by-brick. People who take melatonin at this time are facing a lot of unknowns. Even we researchers have questions about how to use it."

The conservative course of action is to refrain from

taking melatonin at the present time. In five years, we should know a great deal more about the possible benefits and risks of taking the hormone, especially in regard to treating insomnia, biological rhythm disorders, and cancer, which are the most active areas of research at this time. As you wait for the results of these studies, you can focus on preserving and enhancing your natural melatonin supply by following the suggestions made in the previous chapters. If you are in good health and 40 years old or younger, this may be the wisest course of action.

If you are 40 or over, however, or are suffering from one of the diseases or conditions that could be aided by melatonin therapy, you may not want to wait for the research community to provide the data. What is known at the present time about the safety and efficacy of taking the hormone?

MELATONIN IS NONTOXIC

More than three thousand people have taken melatonin in carefully monitored clinical trials. Without exception, these studies have shown that melatonin has little or no toxicity, even in doses as high as several grams taken daily for as long as a month. This dose is thousands of times greater than is required to maintain youthful levels of the hormone. I have colleagues who have taken high doses of melatonin (75 milligrams and up) for ten years or more. The following comments from various researchers and leaders in the pharmaceutical industry attest to the relative safety of melatonin:

There have been no reported cases of acute toxicity from melatonin. The doses that have been ingested have caused blood levels a hundred thousand times higher than naturally occurs.

Robert Sack, M.D., Department of Psychiatry,
Oregon Health Sciences University[1]

One of the nice things about melatonin, from a purely toxicological point of view, is that it is extraordinarily safe.

> Steven Paul, M.D., Vice-President for Drug Discovery,
> Eli Lilly

The amount of melatonin we gave to our patients, one gram per day, was enormous. . . . These large amounts administered for one month produced no apparent toxicity other than drowsiness in any of the subjects. Others have noted the non-toxicity of melatonin.

> Aaron Lerner, M.D., Department of Dermatology,
> Yale University[2]

These observations suggest that the potential therapeutic use of melatonin as an hypnotic [sleep aid] or in the treatment of jet leg is not complicated by undesirable endocrine effects.

> James Wright, Ph.D., University of Surrey, U.K.[3]

We have demonstrated that serum melatonin levels can be maintained at very high levels in melanoma [cancer] patients without significant toxicity.

> M. A. Kane, M.D., Division of Medical Oncology,
> University of Colorado Health Sciences Center[4]

None of the volunteers complained of any adverse reaction apart from a transient increase of evening drowsiness.

> Massimo Terzolo, M.D., San Luigi Hospital, Turin, Italy[5]

No cardiac, hematologic, hepatic, renal or metabolic toxicity was seen in any case during melatonin treatment. Moreover, no undesirable subjective effects were reported. In contrast, most of the patients experienced a relaxation after melatonin injection.

> Paolo Lissoni, M.D., Radiology Division,
> San Gerardo Hospital, Monza, Italy[6]

A substance can have little or no toxicity, however, and still produce negative effects in some people or under some circumstances. In fact, melatonin's very *assets* could turn into liabilities. Consider melatonin's wonderful sleep-enhancing effect. It could prove a decided liability if you were foolish enough to take a high dose of melatonin before driving a car or operating a dangerous piece of machinery.

Another reason to be cautious about taking melatonin is that there is great biological diversity among human beings. Melatonin has not been administered to enough people or for a long enough period of time to rule out the possibility that some people may react atypically to the hormone. In fact, it is possible that some diseases and conditions might be *exacerbated* by melatonin. In this chapter I list some groups of people who may be wise to avoid taking melatonin, but I make no claim that this list is all-inclusive.

In order to uncover all the possible negative side effects of melatonin in the greater population, the hormone would have to be tested in a large, long-term, double-blind, placebo-controlled trial. No such study has been done, and to my great regret, none is likely to be conducted in the near future because there is little financial incentive to investigate a nonpatentable substance. Until a major study is conducted, some will always doubt the safety and efficacy of taking exogenous melatonin for prolonged periods of time.

This said, it must be acknowledged that millions of people are now taking medications with scores of *known* negative side effects, some of them life-threatening. The widely sold pain-reliever acetaminophen is just one example. A study at the Johns Hopkins University revealed that "arthritis sufferers and others who take acetaminophen every day for a year increase their risk of kidney failure about 40 percent."[7] This risk, however, has not stopped people from taking these pain-relievers.

CONTRAINDICATIONS

I am frequently asked, "Are there any people who should *not* take melatonin?" When it comes to medications or food supplements of any nature, even ordinary vitamin supplements, I believe it is best to err on the side of caution. Thus, some people would be wise to refrain from taking melatonin, or to take it only under the close supervision of a physician. On the following pages I have compiled a list of some of those people. I want to emphasize that, for the most part, this list is composed of *theoretically possible* negative side effects, not *known* negative side effects. In the several years that melatonin has been freely available in stores and used by hundreds of thousands of people, I am aware of no reports of serious side effects other than what a major retailer of melatonin calls "occasional individual reactions of a minor and idiosyncratic nature."[8]

CATEGORY OF PERSONS	THEORETICAL RISK
People taking steroid drugs such as cortisone and dexamethasone	Melatonin may counteract the effect of these medications.[9]
Pregnant women	Melatonin has not been tested in pregnant women. Unknown risks.
Women wanting to conceive	Doses greater than 10 milligrams may prevent ovulation in some women.[10]
Nursing mothers	Small amounts of melatonin are transmitted through breast milk.[11]
People with severe mental illness	In an early study, giving massive doses of

	melatonin in the daytime to patients with severe mental illness exacerbated their symptoms.[12]
People with severe allergies	Melatonin stimulates the immune system and could exaggerate an allergic response.[13]
People with autoimmune diseases	Melatonin stimulates the immune system and could exaggerate an autoimmune response.[14]
People with immune-system cancers such as lymphoma and leukemia	Melatonin may further stimulate the immune cells.[15]
Normal children of all ages	Most children have naturally high levels of melatonin. The effects of exogenous melatonin are not known except in the cases of some children suffering from certain mental and physical handicaps who have benefited a great deal from melatonin.[16]

ATYPICAL REACTIONS

A very few people seem to have atypical reactions to taking melatonin. They have insomnia, nightmares, or dream so vividly that they feel as if they're not sleeping. One person reported his experience with melatonin as "virtual sleeping." According to Dr. Stephen Levine, director of

Allergy Research Group (one of the first distributors of melatonin), this reaction also occurred with tryptophan, which was used as a sleep aid and pain-relieving medication before it was taken off the market. "Some people, a few percent, were *stimulated* by tryptophan," says Levine. "There is great genetic variability among humans. We see the same atypical reaction with melatonin and in about the same proportion."[17]

If you are one of the few people who experience this atypical reaction, talk to your physician about what might be causing it. Also, check to see if the preparation you are taking contains anything other than melatonin. Some preparations contain vitamin B-6, and some people who take that particular vitamin late at night report that it makes them feel alert or even agitated. A good friend of mine has this reaction. She has chronic sleep problems and was hoping that melatonin would help her wake up fewer times at night. She bought a bottle of 3-milligram tablets in a formulation that included vitamin B-6. She took one tablet just before going to bed. To her surprise, she had one of her worst nights in decades, getting only one or two hours of sleep.

I suggested to her that she try a tablet that did not contain vitamin B-6 and also take a lower dose of melatonin. She switched to a 1-milligram capsule produced by a different company and had the opposite reaction, sleeping better than she had in a long time. (Note: Many people take the vitamin B-6 preparation with no ill effects.)

THE QUESTION OF CONTAMINATION

Another note of caution is that there is always a possibility of contamination during the manufacture of any drug or food supplement, especially when it is not being regulated by the FDA. A substance with no known toxicity in its pure form could cause a negative reaction if mingled with toxic impurities.

Distributors of vitamins and food supplements have become much more vigilant about assuring the purity of their products, partly because of the tryptophan tragedy discussed in Chapter 16. For example, many companies now conduct their own quality-control tests in addition to demanding a certificate of purity from their wholesalers. One safeguard is to purchase melatonin from companies that have developed a reputation for quality and are taking the added precaution of conducting their own assays. The safest product may not be the cheapest product. (In the Resources section on pages 269–73, we list retailers who conduct independent assays of their melatonin supply.)

Even if a batch of impure melatonin were to appear on the market, however, it is unlikely that people would suffer the severe negative health effects that were associated with the contaminated tryptophan because melatonin is taken in much smaller doses. Typically, people were taking 1 to 2 *grams* of tryptophan a day, while the standard dose for melatonin is 0.05 to 10 *milligrams*, a fraction of that amount. The smaller the amount of a substance, the smaller the amount of a possible contaminant (unless, of course, the contaminant is contained in the supposedly "inert" filler).

CHOOSING AMONG DIFFERENT MELATONIN PREPARATIONS

If you decide to take melatonin supplements, you have a choice of a number of different preparations. Currently, you can buy synthetic melatonin or melatonin that is marketed as a "natural" pineal extract. I urge you to buy the *synthetic* preparation. First of all, tablets that derive their melatonin exclusively from pineal extracts could not contain significant amounts of melatonin. To produce as little as one milligram of pure melatonin, the manufacturer would have to purify the glands of hundreds of thousands of animals. (If you recall, Aaron Lerner estimated he would have to purify the pineal glands of one million cattle to produce 10 milligrams of pure melatonin.) Second, if these tablets contain actual brain tissue, they could contain latent viruses or proteins that might evoke an antibody response.

A safer bet is to purchase synthetic melatonin. High-quality synthetic melatonin is manufactured from pharmaceutical-grade raw materials. Through a complicated series of steps, chemists create a product that is identical in all respects to the melatonin produced by your pineal gland. Synthetic melatonin is the real McCoy.[18]

You can buy synthetic melatonin in a number of forms, including a sublingual tablet (a tablet that dissolves in your mouth), an ordinary tablet or capsule, or a tablet or capsule supplemented with vitamins and herbs. Slow-release tablets are now on the market, and a transmucosal patch (a patch that adheres to your gums) is under investigation. (The transmucosal patch is likely to be available only by prescription.)

The method of delivery can make a significant difference in how much melatonin enters your bloodstream, how fast it gets there, and how long it stays. Most tablets and gelatin capsules are regarded as "fast-release" preparations because no steps have been taken to slow down the rate of absorption. When you swallow a fast-release preparation, it goes to your stomach, where it is broken down into smaller fragments. It then passes from the stomach into blood vessels in the wall of your stomach; this blood is then filtered through the liver. The liver metabolizes a high percentage of the melatonin, converting it into a substance called 6-hydroxymelatonin sulfate, which is then excreted in the urine.[19] (This process is called a first-pass effect, because it is the first time melatonin is presented to the liver.) The amount metabolized on this first pass varies greatly from person to person. A person with an efficient liver may metabolize most of the melatonin, preventing 95 percent of it from entering the general circulation. A person with a less efficient liver may experience a minor first-pass effect, allowing much greater amounts to enter the bloodstream. One study of five individuals found a thirty-fivefold difference in the amount of melatonin in the serum following ingestion of the same 2-milligram dose.[20]

My wife and I, for example, may well metabolize melatonin very differently. She is a petite woman, about half my body weight. And yet when we take the same dose of melatonin, I feel far sleepier than she does. This reaction suggests that more of the hormone makes it through my liver intact, more than offsetting our difference in body size.

At the present time researchers have no way of predicting whose liver is going to metabolize melatonin efficiently and whose is not. The saving grace is that melatonin is nontoxic in high concentrations. Even if you take a small amount of melatonin and wind up with high blood levels of the hormone, the only negative consequence is likely to be next-day drowsiness. If you react in this fashion, simply reduce the dose. Some people take as little as 0.1 milligram a night.

When you take one of these fast-release tablets, you will get peak levels of melatonin in your bloodstream in thirty to sixty minutes. The initial concentration may be very high. Even if you take a small dose (1 to 2 milligrams), you can have melatonin levels in the tens of thousands of picograms per milliliter, far greater than the 50 to 150 picograms normally present in your bloodstream at night. In a fast-release preparation it is necessary to have this initial high concentration because melatonin has a very short half-life, only thirty to sixty minutes. (This means that it takes less than an hour for half of the melatonin that you ingest to disappear from your bloodstream.) You have to start out with a high concentration to keep the amount in your bloodstream sufficiently high throughout the night. The higher the initial concentration of the hormone, the longer it will stay in your bloodstream.

Slow-release (also called timed-release or sustained-release) tablets are now on the market. These products release melatonin in small increments throughout the night, more closely resembling the body's mode of operation. With slow-release preparations, you do not need a high initial surge of the hormone to produce elevated levels throughout the night. This may be the best preparation all around because it allows you to take a smaller dose and also mimics the body's own actions. Slow-release tablets may be especially beneficial for those who awaken in the middle of the night and have problems going back to sleep—melatonin will be there when they need it. (Regular tablets can be metabolized so quickly that if taken at bedtime, most of the hormone may be out of the general circulation by three A.M.)

Sublingual preparations—tablets designed to be dissolved in the mouth—allow a higher percentage of the melatonin to enter the bloodstream. This is because a portion of the melatonin is absorbed through the mucous membranes and enters the blood directly, bypassing the liver and its first-pass effect. The melatonin also gets into your circulation more quickly. If you have difficulty falling asleep, you may want to try a sublingual preparation because you will have higher blood levels of melatonin in a shorter amount of time.

HOW MUCH SHOULD YOU TAKE?

There's no simple answer to the question "How much should I take?" It depends on your age, your reason for taking melatonin, your current melatonin levels, the kind of preparation you use, and how efficiently your liver metabolizes the hormone. To make matters even more complicated, researchers have yet to determine optimum doses for most uses. This is a very young clinical science.

Yet, some overall recommendations have been made. The physicians I've met who prescribe melatonin are in agreement that their patients should take the smallest dose that gives the desired effect. For anti-aging and anti-oxidant purposes, the current consensus is that one should aim at recreating the nighttime levels of a young adult, which is approximately 100 to 150 picograms of melatonin per milliliter. Ideally, one should work with a physician who has the ability to monitor one's nighttime melatonin levels and tailor the dose so that it replicates youthful levels. Lacking this support, they suggest that you take a very small dose—as little as 0.1 milligram. (You may have to subdivide a 1-milligram tablet.)

CURRENTLY RECOMMENDED RANGE OF DOSES

SLEEP: 0.2-10 milligrams, taken at bedtime
JET LAG: 1-10 milligrams taken just before bedtime, local time
ANTI-AGING: 0.1-3 milligrams, taken at bedtime
SHIFT WORK: 1-5 milligrams, taken at beginning of subjective sleep time
IMMUNE STIMULATION: 2-20 milligrams, as recommended by your physician

---

Unless advised otherwise by your physician, take the melatonin close to the time you normally go to sleep. If you take it at approximately the same time every night, say ten or eleven P.M., you will be helping to stabilize and reinforce your biological rhythms, which *in itself* may have an anti-aging effect.[21]

To relieve symptoms of jet lag, take 5 milligrams an hour or so before bedtime, local time, when you reach your new destination. Continue to take a tablet each night until you no longer feel the effects of jet lag. Some people take as much as 10 milligrams, and others do well on as little as 1 milligram. You will need to tailor the dose to your specific physiology.

For sleep purposes, the range of effective doses is extremely wide, from 0.1 milligram to 50 milligrams. Begin by taking 1 to 2 milligrams and increase or decrease the dose as necessary. The highest dose currently being recommended is 10 milligrams. Doses higher than this may result in such high levels of melatonin that your blood levels will remain elevated well into the next day. (In many people, 10 milligrams will cause elevated blood levels for about twelve hours, which is similar to the pineal gland's own nocturnal schedule.)

Those of you who want to use melatonin as an immunotherapy for cancer, AIDS, or other diseases; or to counteract the toxic effects of radiation or chemotherapy; or to lower your blood pressure or cholesterol, please refer your physician to the studies listed in the Notes and References sections. These uses of melatonin are yet investigational and require the close supervision of a knowledgeable medical professional.

WHAT TIME OF DAY AND HOW OFTEN SHOULD YOU TAKE MELATONIN?

Do not take melatonin during the day unless you are a shift worker or are advised to do so by your physician. Normally, the amounts of melatonin in your bloodstream during the daytime are barely measurable. The goal of taking supplements is to augment the body's natural processes, not work at cross-purposes to them. Increasing your daytime levels of melatonin may disrupt your circadian rhythms and cause other undesirable side effects as well. It could also slow your reaction time and increase your risk of accidental injury.

How often should you take melatonin? It depends on your reason for taking the hormone. For chronic insomnia and anti-aging purposes, melatonin is taken every night. Jet lag sufferers take melatonin as long as they are experiencing symptoms, which may be only two or three days. Shift workers take melatonin as needed. Women with

PMS begin taking melatonin at midcycle and continue taking it until the second or third day of menstruation. Some people take melatonin on an occasional basis, such as when they are under unusual stress, feel ill, have a bout of insomnia, or are exposed to a cold or flu virus (but almost *always* at night).

WHAT BENEFITS CAN YOU EXPECT FROM TAKING MELATONIN?

What positive changes can you expect from taking melatonin? A majority of people report that they sleep better the very first night they take it. (Even those without sleep problems report they get a better night's sleep.) Many people discover they get fewer colds and other illnesses. Some report that they seem to heal from injuries more quickly. Some chronic pain sufferers can cut down on their pain medications. A number of people have reported lower cholesterol, blood pressure, or blood glucose levels.

A significant percentage of those who take melatonin experience a noticeably improved mood. Perhaps 1 or 2 percent feel so much better that they have what can only be described as a euphoric experience. Just recently I received a call from a very kind gentleman who told me that melatonin had dramatically improved his life. "I'm not exaggerating when I say that the first night I took melatonin, I knew for the first time what it meant to sleep," he told me. "Before, I would sleep, but it was like I stayed right at the surface. I would dream terrible dreams all night long. When I woke up, I felt so tired and disoriented that I would dread getting out of bed. Now, it's like I have a new life. I'm happier. Easier to be with. Things don't irritate me as easily. I can work under pressure. I only wish I had found melatonin earlier. I have wasted a good part of my life."

Several people have come to see me personally just to say how much better they feel after taking melatonin. The other day a man came to the lab to thank me for appearing on a local TV show to talk about melatonin. He had tried melatonin and felt like a changed person. For him, the greatest benefit was relief from crushing anxiety. "The morning used to be the worst time for me," he said. "I would wake up and experience something very close to a panic attack. I would tell myself to breathe deeply, to hold on, that I would survive. Eventually my anxiety would diminish, and I could get up and begin the day. This doesn't happen with melatonin. I wake up *anticipating* what I'm going to do that day."

In the paragraphs that follow, I have included comments from a number of people about their positive experiences with melatonin. Testimonials such as these are regarded as "anecdotal evidence" and given little weight because there is no way of knowing if the benefits people are reporting are caused by melatonin, the placebo effect, or by some other change in their lives. Controlled studies provide the most reliable data. However, I also find it instructive to hear what people have to say in their own words.

Bonnie T., 76. *"I have diabetes, and I measure my blood glucose twice a day. After I started taking melatonin, my blood glucose levels went down, especially in the afternoon. Also, and I don't know if this is related to melatonin, when I get up in the morning, I feel more sure-footed. My feet feel more flexible, and I walk with more energy. Then I had these dark spots on my chest, and they're fading. That surprised the heck out of me. So I'm really tickled."*

Crystal E., 30. *"I have endometriosis, which gives me painful menstrual cramps, and I've been taking Propaset and Toradol to relieve the pain, but they interrupted my sleep and gave me nightmares. When I started taking melatonin, I no longer had to take the Propaset. I sleep more soundly, have less pain, and no more nightmares."*

Jane R., 47. *"I've been taking melatonin for two years, and I haven't been sick once in that entire time. Not even a cold. I may feel a cold coming on, but it never catches hold. Both my husband and two daughters have had lots of colds. I used to have colds that lasted for weeks. Also, now I sleep better."*

Daniel C., 52. [Daniel is a personal friend of mine and a research scientist. He's been taking melatonin for twenty years.] *"The few times I stopped taking melatonin, I caught a cold and felt tired. So I started taking it again."*

Cheryl S., 48. *"Sometimes I get so wound up I find it hard to sleep. When I take melatonin, I just relax and drift off to sleep."*

Martha K., 63. *"My husband and I both take melatonin. We sleep longer hours. I used to be restless in the night. I'm not now, unless there's some high level of stress in my life. When I do sleep, it's a good sleep, and I feel refreshed after fewer hours. Six hours and sometimes I'm ready to get up and that's fine. It's hard to get my husband to admit how much he's improved. But he sleeps better. Neither one of us gets up as often to go to the bathroom. A lot of nights we don't get up at all."*

Karen H., 50. *"I had elective surgery on both breasts. First one, then a month later the other. In between the two operations, I started taking melatonin. I recovered from the second surgery in half the time than I did from the first."*

Kathryn S., 62. *"For decades I used to wake up at four in the morning and be unable to go back to sleep. Then I'd be tired the next day. Now, with melatonin, I sleep through the night. And my energy lasts throughout the day."*

PART III

▼

THE FUTURE OF MELATONIN RESEARCH

CHAPTER 18

▼

WHEN GOD HOLDS
THE PATENT

Early in my long career as a melatonin researcher, a number of my colleagues questioned my decision to stay in such a "narrow" field of inquiry. Surely I would exhaust my interest and move on to more mainstream research, they supposed. A few people strongly urged me to do so. "Russ, you're seeing stars," they told me in so many words. "Find something more worthy of your time and effort."

The reason I ignored their well-intentioned advice is that there was always one more experiment I had to do to satisfy my curiosity. I would complete that one experiment, only to find another, equally intriguing experiment beckoning me. That study, in turn, suggested another. I was like a child following a trail of crumbs into the forest. Today I have a lot of company. Hundreds of researchers have followed their own trail of crumbs and wound up in the very same woods. Whether their initial interest was cardiology, cancer, epilepsy, sleep, or depression—their search led them, eventually, to melatonin.

With so many scientists now involved in melatonin research, the insights are coming at a very fast pace. At the present time, for example, the NIH is funding 138 separate projects involving melatonin, with more waiting in the wings. I get calls every week from researchers in other fields seeking basic information. This final chapter gives you a preview of where some of this activity may be headed.

As I outlined this chapter, I had a wealth of promising new areas of research to choose from. I could have featured melatonin's potential to treat migraine, protect the developing fetus from fetal alcohol syndrome, delay the onset of neurodegenerative disorders, reduce free-radical damage from oxygen therapy, protect our combat troops from radiation and chemical warfare, or any of a dozen other projects that are now under way or being discussed. But to make this chapter a manageable size, I winnowed my choices down to four—melatonin's ability to treat or prevent autism, sudden infant death syndrome, epilepsy, and diabetes.

By presenting yet more evidence of how melatonin might enhance human health and well-being, I know I am running a risk. Some people are skeptical of melatonin precisely because the hormone has so many potential uses. They imply that melatonin is being touted as a "cure-all," and argue that no one substance is going to insure completely our health and longevity.

I hope I have made it clear throughout this book that melatonin "cures" very little. For example, the hormone shows great promise for strengthening the immune system of AIDS patients, I have explained, but it does not eradicate the disease. It appears to be a wonderful complement to current treatments for cancer, but alone it may have limited effectiveness. Melatonin is a superlative sleep aid, but it does not solve the sleep problems of all people. What we have discovered in the past forty years is that melatonin plays a pivotal role in human physiology, and that the judicious use of the hormone—often in conjunction with other therapies—has the potential to prevent or alleviate a number of conditions. Is it a cure-all? No. But it is clearly one of the most remarkable substances that we produce in our bodies, and deserves all the attention it is getting.

AUTISM

Melatonin is regarded as an anti-aging hormone, and so far most of its clinical applications seem best suited for people 40 and over. Yet melatonin also has the potential to improve the lives of children with various neurological diseases, including autism and epilepsy.

Autism is a devastating disease that afflicts more than 260,000 of our nation's children. The medical dictionary describes autism as "unresponsiveness to human contact, gross deficits in language development, and bizarre responses to various aspects of the environment."[1] Robert and Gay Tesh looked up the definition eight years ago when they were told that their three-year-old son, Michael, was showing typical signs of autism. The symptoms were subtle at first, but they became progressively more noticeable as the years went by. By the time Michael was eight, he was displaying most of the characteristic traits of the disease, including self-destructive behavior. Says his father, "He was biting himself, spinning around compulsively, choking himself. We called it a good day when he spent less than fifty percent of his time in those behaviors."

Michael also had severe sleep difficulties, which are common among autistic children. Robert and Gay would put Michael to bed around eight at night, but he would wake up about two hours later and then stay awake until three or four in the morning. When Michael was awake, he'd disrupt the whole household. Says Robert, "He'd be hyper. Pacing back and forth. We found that taking him for a ride in the car would settle him down, so on the bad nights one of us would drive him around town for forty-five minutes or an hour, and sometimes he'd fall asleep."

The Teshes tried the whole gamut of prescription drugs recommended for autistic children, but nothing seemed to work. Some drugs reduced Michael's hyperactivity, but they made him "cognitively dull. He'd just sit and tune out." Other drugs gave him severe mood swings. Antihistamines prescribed for sleep caused him to have explosive rages.

Meanwhile, Michael began to function less and less well. "Language became very difficult for him," says Robert. "You'd say to him, 'Pick up the toy.' And he'd stand in front of the toy and echo what you had said without comprehension: 'Pick up the toy. Pick up the toy.' English was like a foreign language for him. He became incontinent. You could hold him and try to comfort him, and the next thing you knew, you were being bitten. Pretty severely. I hate to say it, but it was hell." Gay says, "The doctors empathized and sympathized with us, but they had little else to offer."

Like the parents in the movie *Lorenzo's Oil*, Robert and Gay began their own crusade to solve Michael's problems. Using their home computer, Robert searched the medical databases for information relating to autism. When he found a treatment that seemed safe and effective, he would scout out a doctor familiar with the procedure and ask for advice. Some of the therapies they tried made Michael much worse. "We tried a homeopathic remedy, and it had the opposite effect from the one intended. Michael went berserk. He went ballistic." But some of their efforts were rewarded. Among other things, they found a medication that greatly diminished Michael's self-destructive behavior.

But nothing seemed to help Michael sleep—until they discovered melatonin. One of Robert's colleagues had used melatonin as a sleep aid and told him where to buy it. Robert asked a researcher for advice. "There's no harm in trying," he was told.

That very day, Robert and Gay purchased a bottle of melatonin at a local store and decided to give some to their son. "We put Michael to bed at the regular time. Then we woke him up at ten, just before he would normally wake up on his own, and gave him a three-milligram tablet. To our surprise, he went back to sleep and stayed asleep until four A.M. The next night we gave him the melatonin at his normal bedtime, and it kicked right in. He slept through the night. We were ecstatic." They gave melatonin to Michael every night, and the boy continued to sleep through the night.

This reprieve alone was a godsend, but the hormone caused other improvements as well. "His mood got better," says his father, "and he seemed to be able to process information faster. Autistic children have a slow reaction time. It used to be that when we asked Michael a question, we would get an answer twenty minutes later. With melatonin, he began to respond much faster." Whether this was the result of his improved sleep or a more direct effect of melatonin, they did not know.

So thrilled were the Teshes with Michael's progress that they told other parents with autistic children about melatonin. Says Gay, "They'd try melatonin, and then they'd call the next day and say, 'My God! This really works!'" Soon thirty families were giving melatonin to their children.

"All of the kids were sleeping better," says Robert, "and as was true for us, the parents saw other improvements as well. Several children had a reduction in seizure activity. Many children had fewer compulsive behaviors. In general, the children seemed more 'tuned in' to their surroundings."

One child's response was quite dramatic. For seven years, the boy had been obsessed with a yellow kitchen strainer. He played with it incessantly, holding it in his hands and looking at it from all angles. If he couldn't find the strainer, he would panic and not let anyone rest until it was found. As soon as he was reunited with the strainer, he would hold it lovingly and begin humming to himself.

His mother says, "Three weeks after going on melatonin, he lost all interest in the strainer. It became just another object in the house. It sits where he last left it. He seems more interested in people now."

Partly due to the dedication and persistence of Robert and Gay Tesh, researchers at Yale University are now contemplating studying the relationship between autism and melatonin. Meanwhile, at another university, a researcher is beginning to examine the pineal glands of deceased autistic adults. In the summer of 1995 a group of Italian researchers reported that autistic children do not produce the normal nighttime surge of melatonin, implying that a deficiency of melatonin may be a part of the complex neurological disorder.[2]

Despite the many links between melatonin and autism, Robert Tesh is quick to point out that the hormone has not been a miracle cure. "None of the children who are being given melatonin have become normal children. But it does seem to go a long way in controlling their abnormal behaviors. Our son is now doing very well. We've reduced the amount of melatonin we give him, and we no longer give it every night. His health is good. He sleeps well. And overall, I'd say he doesn't broadcast the symptoms that say 'autism.' A casual observer might think he is somewhat retarded—which, believe me, is a big improvement. What pleases us most of all is that, with melatonin, we are able to care for him at home."

EPILEPSY

The trail of evidence demonstrating melatonin's anticonvulsive properties leads back more than thirty years. Decades ago, a number of scientists observed that removing the pineal gland from gerbils can trigger epileptic seizures.[3] Other researchers found that melatonin lowers the excitability of individual neurons and acts as a mild anticonvulsant.[4] Perhaps the most telling study was a

1977 animal experiment in which antibodies to melatonin were injected into rats, eliminating their natural supply of the hormone. Immediately—in fact, in some instances while the injection was still being administered—the animals went into convulsions.[5]

Ferdinando Anton-Tay was the first clinician to administer melatonin to epileptic patients. In 1971 he gave melatonin injections to three epileptic patients. He monitored the brain waves of the patients before and after administering the hormone and found that melatonin normalized their brain waves, particularly during the first four hours after administration.[6] He continued to give melatonin to one of the patients for two additional days, during which time the patient was seizure free, despite the fact that his other medications had been withdrawn.[7]

The most dramatic response to melatonin was observed just recently in a two-year-old Spanish girl named Chiela. Chiela has Lennox-Gastaut syndrome, a form of epilepsy. She was having between fifteen and twenty convulsions a day and was not responding to any form of therapy, including the latest anticonvulsant drugs. Most of the time she was in a coma. Her parents consulted my colleague Dr. Dario Acuña Castroviejo, a professor of physiology at the University of Granada in Spain, who suggested that Chiela be treated with melatonin. She was given an injection of 50 milligrams three times a day. Miraculously, in two days the convulsions stopped. A month later, she appeared almost normal. Today, two years later, she continues to be given melatonin, although in lower doses, and she is virtually symptom free. There is no doubt in the minds of her physicians and parents that melatonin saved Chiela's life.[8]

Interestingly, one way that melatonin may help protect against seizures is by scavenging free radicals. Children who are severely deficient in glutathione peroxidase, one of the key antioxidants in the brain, have been known to have nearly continual seizures. Giving these children selenium (glutathione peroxidase is selenium dependent) has reduced the number of seizures and improved EEG recordings.[9] Melatonin may act in a similar manner. As a potent antioxidant in its own right, as I mentioned earlier, melatonin may also stimulate the activity of gluathione peroxidase in the brain. In any case, the relationship between melatonin and epilepsy deserves closer scrutiny than it has received in the past. I hope that more melatonin researchers and neurologists will pursue this area of research.

SIDS—SUDDEN INFANT DEATH SYNDROME

Sudden infant death syndrome (SIDS), or "crib death," is defined as the death of an infant suddenly and without warning, typically during sleep. Throughout the industrialized world, SIDS is the leading cause of death of children between one and six months of age. Since 1974 the U.S. government has sponsored an intensive campaign to uncover the cause of SIDS, but it has remained an enigma.

Now there is some suggestion that a deficiency of melatonin may be involved in the disorder. Consider these facts: (1) SIDS is classified as a sleep disorder; (2) it has a circadian rhythm, occurring most often at night; and (3) it has a seasonal rhythm, peaking in the winter. The one part of the body that is intimately associated with sleep, circadian rhythms, and seasonal adaptation is the pineal gland.

But the link between SIDS and the pineal gland goes beyond these general observations. Larry Sparks, Ph.D., associate professor of neurology and pathology at the University of Kentucky, has examined the pineal glands of more than a hundred SIDS babies. He reports that in all but a few instances, the glands were small and abnormal in appearance.[10]

Sparks became interested in the role of the pineal gland in SIDS by chance. Several years ago, he was studying the physiology of the human pineal gland. To gather more information, he began examining the brains of infants.

During one particular week, he had four brains available for dissection, two from SIDS babies and two from babies who had died of other causes. By happenstance, all four babies were of the same sex and had died at the same age. When Sparks looked at the four glands, he could see at once that the pineal glands of the SIDS infants were smaller. Examining the glands under a microscope, he observed marked differences in the cytostructure of the tiny organs, which to him "strongly suggested that the glands weren't working right."

Today, having examined more than a hundred pineal glands from SIDS infants, Sparks claims that the pineal glands of SIDS infants are smaller by 50 to 90 percent. "And this is despite the fact that there is no difference in brain size or overall body weight between babies that died of SIDS and other infants," he adds.[11] There is also evidence that these dysfunctional glands produce less melatonin. Richard Wurtman and colleagues compared melatonin levels in the bodily fluids of infants who had died from SIDS with infants who had died from other causes. SIDS infants had significantly lower levels.[12]

How might an abnormal production of melatonin contribute to SIDS? Based on the insights gathered by Sparks and others, as well as my own awareness of melatonin's neuroprotective ability, a scientifically reasonable theory can be constructed. As the brain of the fetus develops, it has been documented, an abundance of neurons are created—more, in fact, than the infant will need later in life. Some of those neurons degenerate in the first few months of life, as a normal and necessary part of human development; in essence, the brain is being "rewired" to a more mature configuration. Sparks has found evidence to suggest that in SIDS babies, the process of cell death continues longer than desirable.[13] The loss of vital neurons, especially in regions of the brain related to sleep, could cause a child to stop breathing during deep sleep, which is thought to be the principal mechanism of death.

Abnormally low levels of melatonin in the brain could contribute to this continued loss of crucial brain cells.

Most babies start producing melatonin around three or four months of age—about the same time that the rate of nerve death should decline. (This is also the age when a baby begins to have a regular sleep-wake cycle.) Evidence is about to be published showing that melatonin reduces brain cell death. A baby with a dysfunctional pineal gland might not produce enough of the neuroprotective hormone to halt the degeneration of additional brain cells.

This theory warrants further investigation. If prolonged low nocturnal levels of melatonin do indeed contribute to the underlying cause of SIDS, then it would be highly desirable to know the nocturnal melatonin production of vulnerable infants. (It is now possible to determine melatonin levels in saliva, a less invasive procedure than drawing blood.) Infants with unusually low levels of the hormone could be given carefully calibrated supplements by their physicians to bring those levels up to normal. It is within the realm of possibility that Sparks's serendipitous observation about the relative size of the pineal glands of four infants could lead to a preventive treatment for the leading cause of infant death.

DIABETES

Diabetes is a deadly disease. Fifty percent of people diagnosed with insulin-dependent (type I) diabetes before the age of 30 are dead by age 50. Diabetes is also the leading cause of new cases of blindness and is a contributing factor in 50 percent of all heart attacks and an even higher percentage of all strokes.

It was reported in 1986 that people with diabetes may have abnormally low levels of melatonin. An English team headed by Josephine Arendt compared the nocturnal melatonin levels of sixteen diabetics with a group of age-matched healthy volunteers. The diabetics were producing significantly less melatonin. In fact, five of the sixteen diabetics had barely detectable amounts of the hormone.

Diabetics with an accompanying nerve disorder called autonomic neuropathy had a flip-flopped circadian rhythm, producing more melatonin during the day than at night.[14]

Low melatonin levels could contribute to a number of health problems common to diabetics. Many diabetics have sleep difficulties, for example. In one study, 33 percent of a group of diabetics had severe sleep problems, compared with only 8 percent of an age-matched group of nondiabetics.[15] Diabetics also have a high incidence of cataracts, hypertension, high cholesterol, infections, and stroke—diseases that may be caused or exacerbated by free radicals.[16] An inadequate supply of antioxidants is likely to increase the risk of being afflicted by these particular conditions.

▶ MELATONIN PREVENTS DIABETES IN ANIMALS

Melatonin may do more than reduce the side effects associated with diabetes: It may help delay its onset or prevent the disease itself. In Locarno, Georges Maestroni and Ario

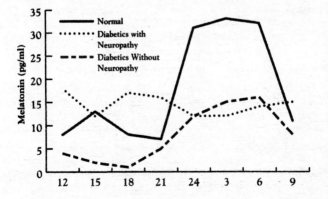

Figure 38. **Diabetics Have Altered Melatonin Rhythms**

Conti are raising a colony of mice that have hereditary diabetes. Typically, 70 percent of the females of this particular strain become diabetic. For the past year, the researchers have been giving half of these mice a nightly dose of melatonin. At the time of my last visit to Locarno, not one of the melatonin-treated mice had come down with the disease. Meanwhile, a high percentage of the mice not being treated with melatonin were showing signs of diabetes. Study results should be available soon. (Maestroni cautions that their findings will apply to type I or insulin-dependent diabetes, not to the more common type II diabetes, which is a metabolic disorder.)

In a previous animal study, melatonin prevented an experimentally induced form of diabetes. When rodents are injected with alloxan, a chemical that generates free radicals, they become diabetic. (The free radicals destroy a part of the pancreas called the islets of Langerhans, which are responsible for producing insulin. This model would also resemble type I diabetes.) In the early 1990s, French researchers discovered that melatonin could block the effects of alloxan. Mice that were injected with melatonin before being exposed to the chemical maintained nearly normal levels of blood sugar, while the mice given alloxan alone developed clear signs of diabetes.[17]

Yet other animal studies have demonstrated a close link between melatonin and diabetes. For example, alloxan has been shown to lower melatonin levels in hamsters.[18] Conversely, when deprived of their normal supply of melatonin, rats develop a diminished production of insulin and high levels of blood glucose. When they are given supplemental melatonin, their insulin function and blood glucose levels return to near normal.[19]

If the lessons learned from these animal studies apply to humans, we may have new hope for diabetics and those at high risk for developing the disease.

OBSTACLES YET TO SURMOUNT

In the nearly forty years since Aaron Lerner solved the riddle of melatonin's chemical structure, the hundreds of scientists researching the molecule have managed to unravel many of its mysteries. Together we have found ways to measure melatonin levels to within a few trillionths of a gram. We have learned how to get accurate, repeatable results from human studies, even though human melatonin production can be influenced by a host of factors, including light levels, electromagnetic fields, the time of day, the time of year, the age of the person, and in women, the menstrual cycle. As we begin to identify the precise manner in which melatonin interacts with the immune system, we are coming one step closer to new immunotherapies for cancer, AIDS, and a host of other diseases. As we explore the nuances of melatonin's role in orchestrating our biological rhythms, we are finding ways to alter those rhythms to help people with circadian rhythm disorders. Most recently, we have gained new insight into what may be melatonin's original and most basic function— protecting organisms from free-radical damage. At long last, these discoveries have begun to come out of the laboratory and into the clinic, helping people live healthier and perhaps even longer lives.

One obstacle remains that we have yet to surmount— the scarcity of funding for melatonin research. Small-scale studies are now being funded, but the large sums needed to fully develop effective melatonin therapies for cancer, AIDS, diabetes, heart disease, and other ills have not been forthcoming. Large studies of this nature are typically funded by pharmaceutical companies who have hopes of bringing a profitable new treatment to market. But no pharmaceutical company has shown a great interest in melatonin research because the molecule cannot be patented.

According to Steven Paul, M.D., vice-president for drug discovery at Eli Lilly, "If you proved melatonin was safe and efficacious but didn't have proprietary rights to it, anybody and his brother could make the compound and sell it." Furthermore, since those other companies would have been spared the enormous expense of research and development, they would be able to sell their own products at a fraction of the cost. "It's a conundrum," agrees Dr. Eric Parker, an executive at Bristol-Myers Squibb. "I don't know how one gets around it. If there is no financial gain in a product, it is basically impossible to convince a drug company to investigate it."

THE FATE OF WAIF DRUGS

This is the state of affairs in an economy where the care of the sick, injured, and elderly is expected to generate a profit. Melatonin, however, is not alone in being bypassed by the pharmaceutical industry. Some other substances are equally unprofitable to investigate, including the so-called orphan drugs, or drugs that treat rare diseases. The customer base for orphan drugs is too small to pay for the cost of research and development. As a humanitarian gesture, the federal government has devised financial incentives to encourage pharmaceutical companies to find treatments for these diseases.

But this legislation is of no use for companies interested in investigating melatonin because the hormone cannot be classified as an orphan drug—it has the potential to help *millions* of people. Yet the lack of patent protection makes it equally unprofitable to research. Instead of investigating melatonin itself, pharmaceutical companies are fabricating "analogues" of melatonin, molecular look-alikes that hopefully share some of the properties of the hormone but are different enough in molecular structure to qualify for a patent. To date, more than a hundred melatonin analogues have been patented.[20] Many more have been developed. Bristol-Myers Squibb, for example, has produced more than a thousand compounds that resemble melatonin.[21]

It is possible that some of these melatonin wannabes will be of great therapeutic value. For example, a compound that had melatonin's sleep-enhancing properties but was metabolized more slowly could prove to be a superior sleep medication. But such a designer drug could have negative or unexpected effects on the human body. When clever chemists work their alchemy—adding "a methoxy substitute at the 8-position of the 2-amidotetralin ring"— they could possibly create a toxic or even cancer-causing compound. The substance would have to undergo extensive animal and human testing. Even so, there is no guarantee that the new drug would not alter our body chemistry in some unforeseen manner. When it comes to safety, I would place my bet on melatonin, which appears to have undergone at least 3 billion years of testing and development.

Furthermore, some of melatonin's many properties may never be equaled. In particular, it may not be possible to produce an analogue of melatonin that has superior or even equivalent antioxidant properties. In our laboratory we have studied molecules very close in structure to melatonin but found that none of them can compare to melatonin's free-radical–scavenging ability. In fact, some molecules that resemble melatonin very closely actually *generate* free radicals.[22] To presume that we can improve on a molecule such as melatonin that may be present in all life-forms may be medical hubris.

I therefore make a simple request: Why not research melatonin itself? Why not devote a hundred million dollars to investigating melatonin's ability to defeat cancer, help the weary sleep better, boost the immune systems of elderly people, and help conquer AIDS? Why not explore the wondrous properties of a natural substance that we produce in our own brains?

To do this research, additional funding must be allocated. But federal funds for medical research of all types are drying up. Grant proposals that receive high ratings from reviewers may be rejected solely because of a lack of money to finance them. For a project that involves a nonpatentable substance such as melatonin, funds from the private sector are almost nonexistent. As a result, researchers must compete tooth and nail to keep their projects alive, a climate that fosters anxiety, greed, and secrecy—states of mind that are antithetical to the pursuit of knowledge. I know a number of talented and dedicated melatonin researchers who could paper their laboratory walls with outstanding but unfunded grant proposals.

To remedy this situation, we may need to revise our policy for financing drug research. One positive step would be to create a new category of drugs that embraces all natural, nonpatentable substances including: (1) hormones such as melatonin; (2) vitamins and minerals; and (3) plant products such as ginkgo biloba, green tea, ginseng, garlic, bananas, papaya extract, rice bran, and oat bran. This category of drugs could be called WAIF drugs—medications that are without any incentive to finance. The nation's lawmakers then need to devise strategies to encourage more investment into WAIF drug research, just as they have for orphan drugs.

The benefits that would come from melatonin research alone, I believe, would more than fund the effort. If melatonin lives up to its promise as a treatment for insomnia, Alzheimer's disease, PMS, jet lag, heart disease, cancer, autism, and AIDS—just to name a few of its potential uses—billions of health care dollars may be saved, not to mention an untold amount of human suffering. With sufficient support from an informed public, I believe we would be able to realize the potential of this wondrous molecule—even though God does indeed hold the patent.

ANSWERS TO COMMON QUESTIONS ABOUT MELATONIN

Since the initial publication of this book, I have received comments and questions about melatonin from hundreds of people. In the following section I have answered some of the most commonly asked questions.

Question: Why do people respond so differently to melatonin? I take a small dose and sleep like a log. My spouse takes three times as much and notices no effect whatsoever.

Answer: Soon after it is absorbed, the melatonin from a tablet or capsule passes through your liver, where some of the hormone is converted into a related substance (6-hydroxymelatonin sulfate), which is then excreted in your urine. Some people have livers that remove most of the melatonin from circulation; as a result, even a relatively high dose of the hormone can have little effect. Others have livers that allow most of it to enter the bloodstream intact, resulting in a noticeable effect from a small dose. The difference among individuals is significant. In one study, five healthy young people took the same 2-milligram dose of melatonin. Among the participants, there was a 35-fold difference in the amount of melatonin that entered the bloodstream.

There is no way of knowing in advance how you will metabolize melatonin, so you may have to find the right dose by trial and error. One physician who prescribes melatonin recommends that you start with a small dose, say 0.5 milligrams, and increase or decrease the dose as necessary. (A dose higher than 10 milligrams may result in high levels of melatonin well into the next day.)

Question: Melatonin helps me fall asleep, but often I wake up in the middle of the night and have a hard time getting back to sleep. Why is this?

Answer: Melatonin has an unusually short half-life, from 30 to 40 minutes. (The term "half-life" refers to the amount of time it takes 50 percent of a given substance to be eliminated from your bloodstream.) This means that several hours after you take melatonin, you may have negligible amounts in your bloodstream, depriving you of its sleep-enhancing effect.

Taking melatonin at bedtime can also *cause* you to wake up very early in the morning, even if you normally sleep soundly throughout the night. This early-morning awakening is caused by the rapid elimination of melatonin from your bloodstream. Normally (that is, without taking supplemental melatonin), the amount of melatonin in your bloodstream falls off around five or six in the morning. This decline in melatonin causes your temperature to rise, which your body interprets as a wake-up signal. When you take supplemental melatonin at bedtime, you create an artificially sharp rise in your melatonin levels for the next few hours and a correspondingly abrupt decline thereafter, causing your body temperature to rise prematurely—which can interrupt your sleep.

People have found various remedies for this problem. Some people take a relatively high dose of melatonin at bedtime, which sustains as elevated level of melatonin throughout the night. (Be wary of taking too much melatonin, however, because you may experience next-day drowsiness.) Others take a second, smaller dose of melatonin if and when they wake up in the middle of the night. A third and increasingly common solution is to take melatonin in a timed-release format. Timed-release preparations release the melatonin gradually throughout the night, preventing a sharp decline in the early morning. A number of timed-release preparations are now on the market.

Question: Will taking melatonin interfere with my body's natural production of the hormone?

Answer: Taking hormonal supplements can cause your body to slow down production of those same hormones, a phenomenon known as a "negative feedback reaction." It is not known for certain whether the prolonged use of melatonin causes such a reaction, but preliminary results from an ongoing clinical trial suggest that it may not. In this trial, 1,400 Dutch women have been taking the B-Oval pill, a preparation that contains a very high dose of melatonin (75 milligrams). The director of the study, Michael Cohen, M.D., Ph.D., reports: "We have not found any problems with prolonged use of melatonin. In particular, we have seen no interference with the endogenous [natural] production of melatonin after long or short use of the hormone. In addition, the women who participated in the trials did not suffer any negative side effects after stopping taking the preparation."

Question: I have heard that melatonin should not be taken by those with an autoimmune disease. I have arthritis. Will I make matters worse by taking melatonin?

Answer: Melatonin has a complex and not fully understood influence on the immune system. It is theoretically possible that taking the hormone might exacerbate an autoimmune disease by stimulating parts of the immune system that are already too reactive.

But there is some preliminary evidence that melatonin may be *helpful* for people with arthritis and certain other autoimmune conditions. It will be years, if not decades, before we have conclusive data. The conservative course of action is to wait for researchers to answer some of these questions or to take melatonin only with the advice and support of a knowledgeable physician.

Question: I've heard that taking melatonin can cause or worsen depression. Is there any truth to this rumor?

Answer: There have been no definitive studies of melatonin's effects on mood. My unofficial survey suggests that it has different effects on different people. Most people say that melatonin has little or no effect on their mood. Some people, however, report that melatonin has worsened their mood, and others claim that it has greatly improved their mood or even relieved long-standing depression. (One man wrote me to say that taking melatonin ended his twenty-year struggle with manic-depression.) Clearly, this area of research deserves more attention. Until we know more about this mercurial molecule, I advise those with a history of depression or mental illness to refrain from taking melatonin or to take it only under the supervision of their doctors.

Question: I'm taking a number of medications. Will melatonin interfere with the positive effects of those drugs or perhaps cause a negative reaction?

Answer: It is possible that melatonin will interfere with some of the actions of steroid drugs. One reason steroid drugs are prescribed is to suppress the immune system, which is a desirable response when treating a number of conditions such as inflammation and various autoimmune disorders. As I've explained in detail earlier in the book, melatonin has a *stimulatory* effect on the immune system. Furthermore, animal studies have shown that it can block the immunosuppressive effect of some steroid drugs. Researchers believe melatonin may also interfere with the immunosuppressive effect of steroids in humans.

There is no evidence that melatonin will counteract the effect of other drugs, however. In fact, melatonin may have a *positive* effect when taken in conjunction with some medications, in particular those drugs that interfere with the body's natural production of melatonin, such as certain pain relievers, heart medications, and sleeping pills. It is possible that melatonin may reduce some of their negative side effects or enhance their effectiveness.

Taking melatonin may also allow people to lower the dosage of some medications. For example, I have heard from a number of diabetics who have found that taking melatonin lowered their blood glucose levels, resulting in a need for smaller insulin injections. Similarly, a number of people with hypertension have told me that melatonin reduced their blood pressure. One woman was able to eliminate one of her two heart medications. A note of caution: Before you add melatonin to other prescription drugs, consult your doctor.

Question: When I take melatonin I have nightmares or sleep less soundly than usual. Why is this?

Answer: A number of people have reported this atypical reaction to melatonin. I am somewhat at a loss to explain this reaction because it has not been observed in any of the clinical trials of melatonin. This suggests to me that the problem may be due to 1) ingredients that may be mixed with the melatonin (for example, many melatonin preparations on the market contain vitamin B-6, which can disrupt sleep); 2) too high a dose; or 3) a "negative placebo effect."

On the other hand, it could be that a minority of people do indeed respond to pure melatonin in an atypical fashion but, by chance, none of them has participated in a clinical trial. It has long been noted that there is great diversity among human beings and that a substance that causes drowsiness in one person can cause insomnia in another.

Whatever the explanation, my letters and phone calls attest to the fact that some people do have restless nights after taking melatonin. Switching to a brand that contains a more pure formulation or lowering the dose has solved the problem for some people. A minority of people have continued to react atypically to melatonin no matter what strategy they try. My advice to them is to stop taking the hormone.

Question: My mother has been diagnosed with terminal cancer. Should she take melatonin?

Answer: Each year, 450,000 people in the United States die from cancer. In their final months, many are plagued with pain, depression, anxiety, insomnia, and/or weight loss. A number of studies have shown that melatonin can prolong the lives of people with terminal cancer and in many instances help improve their quality of life by relieving their pain, improving their mood, reducing the severity of weight loss, and improving their overall physical condition. Melatonin is proving to be a safe, effective, nonaddictive, and inexpensive treatment option for people with advanced cancer. Discuss this with your physician.

Question: How do I know if the melatonin I've purchased is pure and safe?

Answer: Melatonin, like many other substances available in health food stores, is categorized as a food supplement, and producers of food supplements do not have to adhere to the stringent standards mandated for prescription drugs. Therefore, there is less guarantee as to its purity.

As with other food supplements, it is wise to buy melatonin from a company that has earned a reputation for producing quality products—even if the price is somewhat higher. There are several grades of melatonin available for sale. The purer the product, the higher the cost to wholesalers. Melatonin that sells for a bargain basement price may be made from a lesser-grade raw material.

Question: I've been taking melatonin for a number of months and feel stronger and more energetic. I find that I can run faster and farther than before. Is this my imagination, or could it be the result of the melatonin?

Answer: Due to the large number of people now taking melatonin, a number of positive effects have been reported that have yet to be observed in clinical trials. Among them are increased stamina, a relief from dizziness, relief from manic-depression, reduced menstrual pain, shorter and more regular menstrual cycles, less pain from arthritis, and fading of age spots. Whether these responses are coincidental or the direct result of taking melatonin will not be known until controlled studies are conducted.

MELATONIN SURVEY

In order to gather more information about melatonin, we are conducting a survey of melatonin users. Please answer the following questions and mail the information to: Melatonin Survey, 2000 NE 42nd Avenue, Suite 119, Portland, OR 97213. Use as much additional space as you wish. Thank you for your cooperation!

1. How long have you been taking melatonin?

2. Which brand of melatonin are you now taking?

3. What dose and formulation (timed-release, regular-release, sublingual, etc.) are you taking?

4. Does your melatonin preparation contain added ingredients such as vitamins, minerals, or herbs? _____ If so, please list those ingredients.

5. How often do you take melatonin?

6. About what time of day do you normally take melatonin?

7. What is your reason (or reasons) for taking melatonin?

8. What negative effects (if any) have you observed?

9. What positive effects (if any) have you observed?

10. What other comments (if any) would you like to make?

**Visit our internet homepage for updated information about melatonin:
http://www.teleport.com/~jor**

NOTES AND REFERENCES

CHAPTER 2: THE THREE-BILLION-YEAR-OLD MOLECULE

1. Kolaf, J., and Machackova, I. "Melatonin: Does it Regulate Rhythmicity and Photoperiodism Also in Higher Plants?" *Flowering Newsletter* 1994; (17): 53.
2. Poeggeler, B. "Melatonin and the Light-Dark Zeitgeber in Vertebrates, Invertebrates and Unicellular Organisms." *Experientia* 1993; 49: 611–13.
3. Brainard, G.C. "Pineal Research: The Decade of Transformation." *Journal of Neural Transmission* 1978; Suppl 13: 3–10, p. 5.
4. Lerner's insight was that melatonin must be a methoxy derivative of serotonin, an insight that will make sense only to chemists.
5. Melatonin is made from serotonin. In a two-step process, the pineal gland adds enzymes to serotonin to produce melatonin. Even though the two substances are closely related in molecular structure, however, in many cases they have quite opposite effects in the body.
6. Lerner, A.B., and Case, J.D. "Melatonin." *Federation Proceedings* 1960; 19(2): 590–92.
7. Barchas, J., DaCosta, F., and Spector, S. "Acute Pharmacology of Melatonin." *Nature* 1967; 214: 919–20.
8. Anton-Tay, F., Diaz, J.L ., and Fernandez-Guardiola, A. "On the Effect of Melatonin Upon Human Brain.

Its Possible Therapeutic Implications." *Life Sciences* 1971; 10(1): 841–50.

9. The current belief is that the pineal gland continues to produce the same amount of melatonin, but as body mass increases, the concentration in the bloodstream declines.

10. Cavallo, A. "Melatonin and Human Puberty: Current Perspectives." *Journal of Pineal Research* 1993; 15: 115–21.

11. Puig-Domingo, M., Reiter, R., and De Leiva, A. "Brief Report: Melatonin-related Hypogonadotropic Hypogonadism." *New England Journal of Medicine* 1992; 357: 1356–59.

12. Waldhauser, F., Boepple, P.A., and Crowley, Jr., W.F. "Serum Melatonin in Central Precocious Puberty is Lower than in Age-Matched Prepubertal Children." *Journal of Clinical and Endocrinal Metabolism* 1991; 73: 793–96.

13. Puig-Domingo, M., Reiter, R., and De Leiva, A. "Brief Report: Melatonin-related Hypogonadotropic Hypogonadism." *New England Journal of Medicine* 1992; 357: 1356–59.

14. The enzyme is the $[Ca^{2+} + Mg^{2+}]$-dependent ATPase enzyme. We reported on the relationship between melatonin and this enzyme in the following journal article: Chen, L.D. et al. "In Vivo and In Vitro Effects of the Pineal Gland and Melatonin on $[Ca^{2+} + Mg^{2+}]$-Dependent ATPase in Cardiac Sarcolemma." *Journal of Pineal Research* 1993; 14: 178–83.

15. Recent work in our lab has added weight to this theory. We have tested melatonin's antioxidant prowess against closely related molecules, including various metabolites of melatonin. Melatonin has proven superior to each and every one of these contenders. (Serotonin, melatonin's parent molecule, actually *generates* free radicals.) Any organism that came up with a mutant variant of the melatonin molecule would have had a more difficult time surviving, which could be

why the molecule is identical throughout the plant and animal kingdom.

CHAPTER 3: THE BEST ANTIOXIDANT

1. Gutteridge, J.M.C. "Ageing and Free Radicals." *Medical Laboratory Science* 1992; 49: 313–18.
2. Specter, M. "Plunging Life Expectancy Puzzles Russia." *New York Times*, Aug. 2, 1995, p. A1.
3. Some *antioxidants* limit this damage by selflessly replacing the missing electron with one of their own. These antioxidants are called electron donors. Melatonin is an electron donor.
4. Reiter, R.J., Melchiorri, D., Sewerynek, E., Poeggler, B., Barlow-Walder, L.R., Chuang, J.I., Ortiz, G.G., and Acuña-Castroviejo, D. "A Review of the Evidence Supporting Melatonin's Role as an Antioxidant." *Journal of Pineal Research* 1995; 18: 1–11.
5. Tan, D.-X., Poeggeler, B., and Reiter, R.J. "The Pineal Hormone Melatonin Inhibits DNA-Adduct Formation Induced by the Chemical Carcinogen Safrole in Vivo." *Cancer Letters* 1993; 70: 65–71.
6. Vijayalaxmi, B.Z., Reiter, R.J., Sewerynek, E., Meltz, M.L., and Poeggeler, B. "Melatonin Protects Human Blood Lymphocytes from Radiation Induced Chromosome Damage." *Mutation Research* 1995; 346(1): 23–31.
7. Abe, M., Reiter, R.J., and Poeggeler, B. "Inhibitory Effect of Melatonin on Cataract Formation in Newborn Rats: Evidence for an Antioxidative Role for Melatonin." *Journal of Pineal Research* 1994; 17(2): 94–100.
8. Reiter, R.J. "Oxidative Processes and Antioxidative Defense Mechanisms in the Aging Brain." *FASEB Journal* 1995; 9(7): 526–33.
9. Shida, C.S., Castrucci, A.M.L., and Lamy-Freund, M.T. "High Melatonin Solubility in Aqueous Medium." *Journal of Pineal Research* 1994; 16: 198–201.

10. Pieri, C., Marra, M., Moroni, F., and Marcheselli, F. "Melatonin: A Peroxyl Radical Scavenger More Effective than Vitamin E." *Pergamon* 1994; 55(15): 271–76.

11. Reiter, R.J. "Interactions of the Pineal Hormone Melatonin with Oxygen-centered Free Radicals: A Brief Review." *Brazilian Journal of Medical and Biological Research* 1993; 26: 1141–55.

12. Vijayalaxmi, B.Z., Reiter, R.J., Sewerynek, E., Meltz, M.L., and Poeggeler, B. "Melatonin Protects Human Blood Lymphocytes from Radiation Induced Chromosome Damage." *Mutation Research* 1995; 346(1): 23–31.

13. Kahl, R. "Toxicology of the Synthetic Antioxidants BHA and BHT in Comparison with the Natural Antioxidant Vitamin E." *Zeitschrift für Lebensmittel-Untersuchung und -Forschung* 1993; 196(4): 329–38.

14. Menendez-Pelaez, A., and Reiter, R.J. "Distribution of Melatonin in Mammalian Tissues: The Relative Importance of Nuclear Versus Cytosolic Localization." *Journal of Pineal Research* 1993; 15: 59–69.

15. Tan, D.-X., Reiter, R.J., Chen, L.-D., and Barlow-Walden, L.R. "Both Physiological and Pharmacological Levels of Melatonin Reduce DNA Adduct Formation Induced by the Carcinogen Safrole." *Carcinogenesis* 1994; 15(2): 215–18.

CHAPTER 4: BOOSTING THE IMMUNE SYSTEM

1. Meares, A. "Stress, Meditation and the Regression of Cancer." *Practitioner* 1982; 226: 1607–09.

2. Kemeny, M.E., et al. "Repeated Bereavement, Depressed Mood, and Immune Parameters in HIV Seropositive and Seronegative Gay Men." *Health Psychology* 1994; 13(1): 14–24.

3. Stein, M., Miller, A.H., and Trestman, R.L. "De-

pression, the Immune System, and Health and Illness." *Archives of General Psychiatry* 1991; 48: 171–77.

4. Van-Vollenhoven, R.F., and McGuire, J.L. "Estrogen, Progesterone, and Testosterone: Can They Be Used to Treat Autoimmune Diseases?" *Cleveland Clinic Journal of Medicine* 1994; 61(4): 276–84.

5. Bennett, H.T., and Cohen, S. "Stress and Immunity in Humans: A Meta-Analytic Review." *Psychosomatic Medicine* 1993; 55: 364–79. In particular, stress can cause a relative deficiency of circulating B cells, T-helper cells, suppressor/cytotoxic T cells, and natural killer cells.

6. Although I am aware that some of the experiments we conducted were highly stressful to the animals, we rarely kept them long enough to know if there were any effects on their immune system.

7. Maestroni, G.J., Conti, A., and Pierpaoli, W. "Pineal Melatonin, Its Fundamental Immunoregulatory Role in Aging and Cancer." *Annals of the New York Academy of Sciences* 1988; 521: 140–48.

8. Virginia Utermohlen, unpublished study, Cornell University.

9. Neri, B., Brocchi, A., and Cagnoni, M. "Effects of Melatonin Administration on Cytokine Production in Patients with Advanced Solid Tumors." *Oncology Reports* 1995; 2: 45–7.

10. Song, L., Ho Kim, Y., and Adler, W.H. "Age-Related Effects in T Cell Activation and Proliferation." *Experimental Gerontology* 1993; 28: 313–21.

11. Moore, T.J. *Lifespan* (New York: Simon & Schuster, 1993), p. 20.

12. *Journal of Health and Mortuary Statistics* 1995: 4:26–31.

13. Caroleo, M.C., Frasca, D., and Doria, G. "Melatonin as Immunomodulator in Immunodeficient Mice." *Immunopharmacology* 1992; 23: 81–89.

14. Ben-Nathan, D., Maestroni, G.J., and Conti, A., "Protective Effects of Melatonin in Mice Infected

with Encephalitis Viruses." *Archives of Virology* 1995; 140: 223–30.

15. Maestroni, G.J. "T-Helper-2 Lymphocytes as Peripheral Target of Melatonin Signaling." *Journal of Pineal Research* 1995; 18: 84–89.

16. Reiter, R.J., Menendez-Pelaez, A., Poeggeler, B., and Tan, D.-X., "The Role of Melatonin in the Pathophysiology of Oxygen Radical Damage." In *Advances in Pineal Research*, vol. 8, ed. M. Møller and P. Pévet (London: John Libbey and Co., 1994), p.278.

17. Morrey, K.M., McLachlan, J.A., and Bakouche, O. "Activation of Human Monocytes by the Pineal Hormone Melatonin." *Journal of Immunology* 1994; 153: 2671–80.

18. Maestroni, G.J. "T-Helper-2 Lymphocytes as Peripheral Target of Melatonin Signaling." *Journal of Pineal Research* 1995; 18: 84–89.

19. In mice, melatonin caused a significant increase in leukocytes, platelets, and marrow granulocyte/macrophage-colony-forming units. See Maestroni, G.J. "T-Helper-2 Lymphocytes as Peripheral Target of Melatonin Signaling." *Journal of Pineal Research* 1995; 18: 84–89.

CHAPTER 5: NEW HOPE FOR AIDS PATIENTS

1. Kolata, G. "New AIDS Findings on Why Drugs Fail May Shift Research." *New York Times*, Jan. 12, 1995, p. A1.

2. For a clear exposition of this new understanding of HIV, refer to "How HIV Defeats the Immune System" in the August 1995 issue of *Scientific American*, pp. 58–65.

3. Balter, M. "Cytokines Move from the Margins into the Spotlight." *Science* 1995; 268: 205–06.

4. Neri, B., Brocchi, A., and Cagnoni, M. "Effects of Melatonin Administration on Cytokine Production

in Patients with Advanced Solid Tumors." *Oncology Reports* 1995; 2: 45–47.

5. Maestroni, G.J. "The Immunoneuroendocrine Role of Melatonin." *Journal of Pineal Research* 1993; 14: 1–10.

6. Maestroni, G.J. "T-Helper-2 Lymphocytes as Peripheral Target of Melatonin Signaling." *Journal of Pineal Research* 1995; 18: 84–89.

7. Froldi, M., et al. "Mediator Release in Cerebrospinal Fluid of Human Immunodeficiency Virus-Positive Patients with Central Nervous System Involvement. *Journal of Neuroimmunology* 1992; 38(1–2): 155–61.

8. It was discovered that there is a nuclear receptor for melatonin. When melatonin links with this receptor, it down-regulates the expression of 5-lipoxygenase in B lymphocytes about fivefold. This results in a significant reduction in the production of leukotrienes, which play a role in inflammatory diseases such as asthma, inflammatory bowel disease, and arthritis and are known to be high in AIDS patients. See Steinhilber, D., Brungs, M., and Carlberg, C. "The Nuclear Receptor for Melatonin Represses 5-Lipoxygenase Gene Expression in Human B-Lymphocytes." *Journal of Biological Chemistry* 1995; 270(13): 7037–40.

9. Schroder, H.C., et al. "Avarol Restores the Altered Prostaglandin and Leukotriene Metabolism in Monocytes Infected with Human Immunodeficiency Virus Type 1." *Virus Research* 1991; 21(3): 213–23.

10. Tan, D.-X., Chen, L.-D., and Reiter, R.J. "Melatonin: A Potent, Endogenous Hydroxyl Radical Scavenger." *Endocrine Journal* 1993; 1: 57–60.

11. Barlow-Walden, L.R., Reiter, R.J., and Poeggeler, B. *Effects of Melatonin on Brain Glutathione Peroxidase Activity.* (Department of Cellular and Structural Biology, University of Texas Health Science Center, 1995.)

12. Chuang, J.-I., et al. "Inhibitory Effect of Melatonin on NF-κB in Rat Spleen." In press. Interestingly, we discovered that physiological levels of melatonin also inhibit NF-κB binding activity. Rats that were sacri-

ficed at night had a 24 percent reduction in splenic NF-κB binding activity compared with rats sacrificed in the daytime. The difference was attributed to the normal nighttime rise of melatonin.

13. The group consisted of six LAS-ARC and five AIDS patients who were regarded as terminal. There were nine men and three women; their average age was 28.1.

14. Colombo, F. *Melatonina: da marker a farmaco anti invecchiamento.* (University of Pavia, Italy, 1992.)

15. Interestingly, melatonin has been shown to stimulate the production of growth hormone in males. According to a 1993 paper, "Our data indicate that oral administration of melatonin to normal human males increases basal GH release and GH responsiveness to GHRH through the same pathways as pyridostigmine. Therefore it is likely that melatonin plays this facilitatory role at the hypothalamic level by inhibiting endogenous somatostatin release." Valcavi, R., Zini, M., Maestroni, G., and Conti, A. "Melatonin Stimulates Growth Hormone Secretion Through Pathways Other Than the Growth Hormone–Releasing Hormone." *Clinical Endocrinology* 1993; 39: 193–99.

16. Marijuana may stimulate the appetite via its stimulatory effect on melatonin. In Chapter 16, I will explain that marijuana is an extremely effective stimulator of melatonin production.

17. Melatonin has produced a similar response in terminal cancer patients.

18. Ochitill, H., et al. "Psychotropic Drug Prescribing for Hospitalized Patients With Acquired Immunodeficiency. *American Journal of Medicine* 1991; 90(5): 601–05.

19. McIntyre, I., Burrows, G.D., and Norman, T.R. "Suppression of Plasma Melatonin by a Single Dose of the Benzodiazepine Alprozalam in Humans." *Biological Psychiatry* 1988; 24: 105–08.

20. Steinberg, R., and Soyka, M. "Problems in Long-term

Benzodiazepine Treatment." *Schweizerische Rundschau für Medizin Praxis* 1989; 78: 784–87.

21. Maestroni, G.J. "T-Helper-2 Lymphocytes as Peripheral Target of Melatonin Signaling." *Journal of Pineal Research* 1995; 18: 84–89.

22. Georges Maestroni, personal communication.

23. Maestroni, G.J. "Melatonin Regulation of Endogenous T-Cell Derived Hematopoietic Cytokines." *Cancer Research.* 1994; 54: 2429–32. Maestroni has shown that melatonin stimulates GM-CSF, a cytokine that stimulates production of neutrophils, monoytes, and macrophages. Synthetically derived GM-CSF is commonly used to treat bone marrow deficiency following cancer or AIDS chemotherapy. Melatonin stimulates this cytokine naturally.

24. Lissoni, P., Brivio, F., and Barni, S. "Low-Dose Subcutaneous Interleukin-2 Therapy in Association with the Pineal Indole Melatonin in Treating AIDS." In Einhorn, J., Nord, C., and Norrby, S.R., ed., *Recent Advances in Chemotherapy*, Proceedings of the 18th International Congress of Chemotherapy, Sweden, June–July 1993 (Stockholm, Sweden: American Society for Microbiology, 1994), pp. 769–70.

25. The amount of IL-2 being administered was 3×10^6 IU/day.

26. Lissoni, P., Brivio, F., Barni, S. "Low-Dose Subcutaneous Interleukin-2 Therapy in Association with the Pineal Indole Melatonin in Treating AIDS." In Einhorn, J., Nord, C., and Norrby, S.R., ed., *Recent Advances in Chemotherapy*, Proceedings of the 18th International Congress of Chemotherapy, Sweden, June–July 1993 (Stockholm, Sweden: American Society for Microbiology, 1994), pp. 769–70. A peak level of responsiveness was detected after two to three weeks, demonstrating once again the importance of a three-week-on, one-week-off protocol.

27. Maestroni, G.J. "The Immunoneuroendocrine Role of Melatonin." *Journal of Pineal Research* 1993; 14: 1–10.

28. Caroleo, M., Frasca, D., Nistico, G., and Doria, G.

"Melatonin as Immunomodulator in Immunodeficient Mice." *Immunopharmacology* 1992; 23: 81–89.

29. Hadden, J.W. "T-Cell Adjuvants." *International Journal of Immunopharmacology* 1994; 16(9): 703–10.

30. Neri, B., Brocchi, A., Carossino, A., Cini-Neri, G., Gemelli, M., Tomassi, M., and Cagnoni, M. "Effects of Melatonin Administration on Cytokine Production in Patients with Advanced Solid Tumors." *Oncology Reports* 1995; 2: 45–47.

31. Lissoni, P., Barni, S., and Tancini, G. "Efficacy of the Concomitant Administration of the Pineal Hormone Melatonin in Cancer Immunotherapy with Low-Dose IL-2 in Patients with Advanced Solid Tumors Who Had Progressed on Il-2 Alone." *Oncology* 1994; 51: 344–47.

32. Neri, B., Brocchi, A., Carossino, A., Cini-Neri, G., Gemelli, M., Tomassi, M., and Cagnoni, M. "Effects of Melatonin Administration on Cytokine Production in Patients with Advanced Solid Tumors." *Oncology Reports* 1995; 2: 45–47.

33. Fuchs, D., Shearer, G., Boswell, R., Lucey, D., Clerici, M., Reibnegger, G., Werner, E., Zajac, R., and Wachter, H. "Negative Correlation Between Blood Cell Counts and Serum Neopterin Concentration in Patients with HIV-1 Infection." *AIDS* 1991; 5(2): 209–12.

34. Famularo, G., De Simone, C., and Coco, F. "Treatment and Prevention of Mycobacterium Avium Complex Infection in AIDS." *Annali italiani di medicina interna* 1994; 9(4): 249–54.

35. Fan, S.-X., Turpin, J.A., and Meltzer, M.S. "Interferon-gamma Protects Primary Monocytes Against Infection with Human Immunodeficiency Virus Type 1." *Journal of Leukocyte Biology* 1994; 56(3): 362–68.

36. Yahi, N., Spitalnik, S.L., and Fantini, J. "Interferon-gamma Decreases Cell Surface Expression of Galactosyl Ceramide, the Receptor for HIV-1 GP120

on Human Colonic Epithelial Cells." *Virology* 1994; 204(2): 550–57.

37. Tosi, P., Visani, G., Ottaviani, E., Gamberi, B., Cenacchi, A., and Tura, S. "Synergistic Cytotoxicity of ZDV plus Alpha and Gamma Interferon in Chronic Myeloid Leukemia Cell like K562." *European Journal of Haematology* 1993; 51(4): 209–213.

38. Maestroni, G.J. "T-Helper-2 Lymphocytes as Peripheral Target of Melatonin Signaling." *Journal of Pineal Research* 1995; 18: 84–89.

39. Montaner, L.J., and Gordon, S., "Th2 Downregulation of Macrophage HIV-1 Replication." *Science* 1995; 267: 538–39.

40. Montaner, L.J., and Gordon, S., "Th2 Downregulation of Macrophage HIV-1 Replication." *Science* 1995; 267: 538–39.

41. Denis, M., and Ghadirian, E. "Interleukin 13 and Interleukin 4 Protect Bronchoalveolar Macrophages from Productive Infection with Human Immunodeficiency Virus Type 1 ."*AIDS Research and Human Retroviruses* 1994; 10(7): 795–802.

42. Sonoda, Y. "Interleukin-4—a dual regulatory factor in hematopoiesis." *Leukemia and Lymphoma* 1994; 14(3–4): 231–40.

43. Maestroni, G.J. "Melatonin Regulation of Endogenous T-Cell Derived Hematopoietic Cytokines." *Cancer Research* 1994; 54: 2429–32.

44. Goletti, D., Kinter, A., Biswas, P., Bende, S., Poi, G. and Fauci, A. "Effect of Cellular Differentiation on Cytokine-Induced Expression of Human Immunodeficiency Virus in Chronically Infected Promonocytic Cells: Dissociation of Cellular Differentiation and Viral Expression." *Journal of Virology* 1995 ; 69(4): 2540–46.

45. Denis, M., and Ghadirian, E. "Interleukin 13 and Interleukin 4 Protect Bronchoalveolar Macrophages from Productive Infection with Immunodeficiency Virus Type 1." *AIDS Research and Human Retroviruses* 1994; 10(7): 795–802.

46. Scadden, D. "The Use of GM-CSF in AIDS." *Infection* 1992; 20 Suppl. 2: 103–06.

47. Scadden, D.T., Bering, H.A., and Groopman, J.E. "Granulocyte-Macrophage Colony-Stimulating Factor Mitigates the Neutropenia of Combined Interferon Alfa and Zidovudine Treatment of Acquired Immune Deficiency Syndrome-Associated Kaposi's Sarcoma." *Journal of Clinical Oncology* 1991; 9(12): 2235–37.

48. Del Gobbo, V., Libri, V., Villani, R., Calio, R., and Nistico, G. "Pinealectomy Inhibits Interleukin-2 Production and Natural Killer Activity in Mice." *International Journal of Immunopharmacology* 1989; 11: 567–77.

49. Ratcliffe, L.T., Lukey, P.T., and Ress, S.R. "Reduced NK Activity Correlates with Active Disease in HIV Patients with Multidrug-Resistant Pulmonary Tuberculosis." *Clinical Experimental Immunology* 1994; 97(3): 373–79.

50. Huang, X.-L., Fan, Z., and Rinaldo, C. "Enhancement of Natural Killer Cell Activity in Human Immunodeficiency Virus-Infected Subjects by In Vitro Treatment with Biologic Response Modifier OK-432." *Clinical and Diagnostic Laboratory Immunology* 1995; 2(1): 91–97.

51. Mansour, I., Doinel, C., and Rouger, P. "CD16+ NK Cells Decrease in all Stages of HIV Infection through a Selective Depletion of the CD16+CD8+CD3– Subset." *AIDS Research and Human Retroviruses* 1990; 6(12): 1451–57.

52. Colombo, F. *Melatonina: da marker a farmaco anti invecchiamento.* (University of Pavia, Italy, 1992).

53. Taylor, S., et al. "Cells and Mediators Which Participate in Immunoglobulin Synthesis by Human Mononuclear Cells." *Clinical and Experimental Immunology* 1990; 80: 130–35.

54. Maestroni, G.J. "The Immunoneuroendocrine Role of Melatonin." *Journal of Pineal Research* 1993; 14: 1–10.

55. Muller, F., Froland, S.S., and Brandtzaeg, P. "Both

IgA Subclasses Are Reduced in Parotid Saliva from Patients with AIDS." *Clinical and Experimental Immunology* 1991; 83(2): 203–09.

56. Lissoni, P., Barni, S., Frigerio, A.F. "Pineal-Opioid System Interactions in the Control of Immunoinflammatory Responses." *Annals of the New York Academy of Sciences* 1994; 471: 191–96. When melatonin was administered to cancer patients in conjunction with IL-2, the patients had a significant reduction in neopterin levels compared with patients treated with IL-2 alone.

57. Fuchs, D., et al. "Negative Correlation Between Blood Cell Counts and Serum Neopterin Concentration in Patients with HIV-1 infection." *AIDS* 1991; 5: 209–12.

58. Lissoni, P., Barni, S., Frigerio, A.F. "Pineal-Opioid System Interactions in the Control of Immunoinflammatory Responses." *Annals of the New York Academy of Sciences* 1994; 471: 191–96.

59. Harris, P. "Eosinophils and AIDS." *Medical Hypotheses* 1994; 43(2): 75–76.

60. Najean, Y., and Rain, J. "The Mechanism of Thrombocytopenia in Patients with HIV Infection." *Journal of Laboratory and Clinical Medicine* 1994; 123(3): 415–20.

61. Reiter, R.J. "Interactions of the Pineal Hormone Melatonin with Oxygen-centered Free Radicals: A Brief Review." *Brazilian Journal of Medical and Biological Research* 1993; 26: 1141–55.

62. Passi, S., De Luca, C., and Ippolito, F. "Blood Deficiency Values of Polyunsaturated Fatty Acids of Phospholipids, Vitamin E and Glutathione Peroxidase as Possible Risk Factors in the Onset and Development of Acquired Immunodeficiency Syndrome." *Giornale italiano di dermatologia e venereologia* 1990; 125(4): 125–30.

63. Fuchs, J., Schofer, H., Milbradt, R., Freisleben, H., Buhl, R., Siems, W., and Grune, T. "Studies on Lipoate Effects on Blood Redox State in Human Immu-

nodeficiency Virus Infected Patients." *Arzneimittel-Forschung* 1993; 43(12): 1359–62.

64. Favier, A., Sappey, C., Leclerc, P., Faure, P., and Micoud, M. "Antioxidant Status and Lipid Peroxidation in Patients Infected with HIV." *Chemico-Biological Interactions* 1994; 91: 165–80.

65. Suzuki, Y., and Packer, L. "Inhibition of NK-kappa B Activation by Vitamin E Derivatives." *Biochemical and Biophysical Research Communications* 1993; 193(1): 277–83. While it is true that many antioxidants can block NK-kappa beta activation, many of them also inhibit production of T lymphocytes in the doses that are high enough to be effective. (See Aillet, F., Gougerot-Pocidalo, M.A., and Israel, N. "Appraisal of Potential Therapeutic Index of Antioxidants on the Basis of Their In Vitro Effects on HIV Replication in Monocytes and Interleukin-2–Induced Lymphocyte Proliferation." *AIDS Research and Human Retroviruses* 1994; 10: 405–11.) Melatonin does not have this liability. In fact, it has been shown to stimulate T cell proliferation.

66. Coodley, G., Nelson, H., Loveless, M., and Folk, C. "Beta Carotene in HIV Infection." *Journal of Acquired Immune Deficiency Syndromes* 1993; 6(3): 272–76.

67. Malorni, W., Rivabene, R., and Donelli, G. "N-Acetylcysteine Inhibits and Decreases Viral Particles in HIV-chronically Infected U937 Cells." *Federation of European Biochemical Societies* 1993; 327(1): 75–78.

68. Barlow-Walden, L.R., Reiter, R.J., and Poeggeler, B. *Effects of Melatonin on Brain Glutathione Peroxidase Activity* (Department of Cellular and Structural Biology, University of Texas Health Science Center, 1995.)

69. Steinhilber, D., Brungs, M., and Carlberg, C. "The Nuclear Receptor for Melatonin Represses 5-Lipoxygenase Gene Expression in Human B-Lymphocytes." *Journal of Biological Chemistry* 1995; 270(13): 7037–40.

70. Colombo, F. *Melatonina: da marker a farmaco anti invecchiamento*. (University of Pavia, Italy, 1992.)
71. Valcavi, R., Zini, M., Maestroni, G., and Conti, A. "Melatonin Stimulates Growth Hormone Secretion Through Pathways Other Than the Growth Hormone–Releasing Hormone." *Clinical Endocrinology* 1993; 39: 193–99.
72. Zhdanova, I.V., Wurtman, R.J., and Schomer, D.L. "Sleep-inducing Effects of Low Doses of Melatonin Ingested in the Evening." *Clinical Pharmacology and Therapeutics* 1995; 57: 552–58.

CHAPTER 6: TAMING THE SAVAGE CELL

1. The dose of melatonin Starr was using was 1 mg/kg, which in a 150-pound adult would amount to around 70 milligrams. It was given intravenously.
2. DMBA is 7,12-dimethylbenz(∂)anthracene.
3. Tamarkin, L., Cohen, M., and Chabner, B. "Melatonin Inhibition and Pinealectomy Enhancement of 7,12-Dimethylbenz(∂)anthracene-induced Mammary Tumors in the Rat." *Cancer Research* Nov. 1981; 41: 4432–36.
4. Blask, D.E., and Hill, S.M. "Effects of Melatonin on Cancer: Studies on MCF-7 Human Breast Cancer Cells in Culture." *Journal of Neural Transmission* 1986; 21: 433–49.
5. Cos, S., and Sanchez-Barcelo, E.J. "Differences Between Pulsatile or Continuous Exposure to Melatonin on MCF-7 Breast Cancer Cell Proliferation." *Cancer Letters* 1994; 85: 105–09.
6. Amy Langer, personal communication.
7. Cohen M., Chabner B., Lippman M. Role of Pineal Gland in Aetiology and Treatment of Breast Cancer. *Lancet* 1978: 814–16.
8. Michael Cohen, personal communication.
9. Amy Langer, personal communication.

10. "Facts About Breast Cancer in the USA," a fact sheet produced by the National Alliance of Breast Cancer Organizations, Feb. 1995.

11. Also, both estrogen and tamoxifen arrest the growth of the cells at the same stage of development, causing a delay in the progression from the G_1 stage to the S phase of the cell cycle. Cos, S., Blask, D.E., and Hill, S.M. "Effects of Melatonin on the Cell Cycle Kinetics and 'estrogen-rescue' of MCF-7 Human Breast Cancer Cells in Culture." *Journal of Pineal Research*, 1991; 10:36.

12. Wilson, S.T., Blask, D.E., and Lemus-Wilson, A.M. "Melatonin Augments the Sensitivity of MCF-7 Human Breast Cancer Cells to Tamoxifen In Vitro." *Journal of Clinical Endocrinology and Metabolism* 1992; 75(2): 669–70.

13. Lissoni, P., and Barni, S. *British Journal of Cancer* 1995; 71: 001–03.

14. One of the promising findings to emerge from Lissoni's study is that melatonin plus tamoxifen proved effective against two different kinds of breast cancer, "estrogen-positive" and "estrogen-negative" breast cancer. (These designations refer to the number of estrogen receptors on the tumor cells.) Estrogen-negative breast cancer is notoriously difficult to treat. The fact that the new therapy inhibited both cell types is good news indeed.

15. David Blask, personal communication.

16. *Lancet* 1994 Mar. 5; 343: 594.

17. As this book goes to press, neither study has been published.

18. Loeb, S., ed. *Professional Guide to Diseases*. 4th ed. (Springhouse, PA: Springhouse Corp., 1992), p. 1311.

19. Lissoni, P., Barni, S., Tancini, G., and Fraschini, F. "Clinical Study of Melatonin in Untreatable Advanced Cancer Patients." *Tumori* 1987; 73: 475–80.

20. Maestroni and Conti had shown that melatonin plus IL-2 is a more effective anticancer treatment in mice than IL-2 alone.

21. Lissoni, P., Barni, S., and Frigerio, A.F. "Pineal-Opioid System Interactions in the Control of Immunoinflammatory Responses." *Annals of the New York Academy of Sciences* 1994; 741: 191–96.

22. Three million international units.

23. Lissoni, P., Barni, S., Brivio, F., and Maestoni, G.J. "A Randomised Study with Subcutaneous Low-Dose Interleukin 2 Alone vs Interleukin 2 Plus the Pineal Neurohormone Melatonin in Advanced Solid Neoplasms Other Than Renal Cancer and Melanoma." *British Journal of Cancer* 1994; 69: 196–99.

24. Adding melatonin to IL-2 also greatly increased the types of cancers that responded to the treatment. Partial responses were obtained in cancers of the lungs, endocrine glands, brain, colon, stomach, liver, and pancreas.

25. Cisplatin (20mg/m^2) and etoposide (100mg/m^2).

26. Lissoni, P., Meregalli, S., Barni, S., and Frigerio, F. "A Randomized Study of Immunotherapy with Low-Dose Subcutaneous Interleukin-2 Plus Melatonin vs Chemotherapy with Cisplatin and Etoposide as First-Line Therapy for Advanced Non-Small Cell Lung Cancer." *Tumori* 1994; 80: 464–67.

27. Lissoni, P., Barni, S., and Maestoni, G.J. "Immunotherapy with Subcutaneous Low-Dose Interleukin-2 and the Pineal Indole Melatonin as a New Effective Therapy in Advanced Cancers of the Digestive Tract." *British Journal of Cancer* 1993; 67: 1404–1407.

28. There was some evidence that MSH stimulates melanoma, and in many ways, melatonin is MSH's opposite. Also, a variety of test-tube and animal studies had shown that melatonin had the potential to inhibit melanoma cell growth.

29. Kane, M.A., Johnson, A., and Robinson, W.A. "Se-

rum Melatonin Levels in Melanoma Patients After Repeated Oral Administration." *Melanoma Research* 1994; 4: 59–65.

30. Lettko, M. "Vitamin B–Induced Prevention of Stress-Related Immunosuppression." *Annals of the New York Academy of Sciences* 1990; 585: 241–49.

31. Paolo Lissoni, personal communication.

32. These side effects are drawn from the list of adverse reactions included in the brochure provided by the manufacturer of Neupogen.

33. Kolata, G. "Women Rejecting Trials for Testing a Cancer Therapy." *New York Times*, Feb. 15, 1995, pp. A1, B7.

34. Maestroni, G.J., Covacci, V., and Conti, A. "Hematopoietic Rescue via T-Cell-dependent, Endogenous Granulocyte-Macrophage Colony-Stimulating Factor Induced by the Pineal Neurohormone Melatonin in Tumor-bearing Mice." *Cancer Research* 1994; 54: 2429–32. In particular, the treatment caused a highly significant increase in leukocytes, platelets, and GM-CFU.

35. Maestroni, G.J. "T-Helper-2 Lymphocytes as Peripheral Target of Melatonin Signaling." *Journal of Pineal Research* 1995; 18: 84–89. Maestroni made the following remarks in this paper: "Our results suggest that melatonin may rescue bone marrow progenitor cells from the toxic effect of cancer chemotherapy compounds via a two-step cytokine cascade. The first step involves the production of IL4 by Th2 bone marrow cells. The second one involves adherent stromal cells which upon IL4 stimulation release GM-CSF. If injected in normal untreated mice or added in a GM-CFU assay in absence of GM-CSF, melatonin does not show any activity."

36. The doses being administered are 110 mg/m^2 of epirubicin and 700 mg/m^2 of cyclophosphamide. This is a relatively aggressive form of treatment. This information is from personal communication with Pedrazzini.

37. From a poster presented at the Apr. 29–May 3, 1995 meeting of the American Radium Society in Paris. "Radioendocrine Therapy of Brain Malignant Gliomas with Radiotherapy in Association with the Pineal Hormone Melatonin: Preliminary Results." Only five out of the ten patients who received radiation plus melatonin were evaluable at the end of a year.

CHAPTER 7: PROTECTING YOUR HEART

1. Statistics are from the American Heart Association publication "Heart and Stroke Facts," 1995 Statistical Supplement.
2. Steinberg, D. "Clinical Trials of Antioxidants in Atherosclerosis: Are We Doing the Right Thing?" *Lancet* 1995; 346: 36–38.
3. Chen, L.-D., Reiter, R.J., and Poeggeler, B. "In Vivo and In Vitro Effects of the Pineal Gland and Melatonin on $(Ca^{2+} + Mg^{2+})$-Dependent ATPase in Cardiac Sarcolemma." *Journal of Pineal Research* 1993; 14: 178–83.
4. Muller, J., Stone, P., and Braunwald, E. "Circadian Variation in the Frequency of Onset of Acute Myocardial Infarction." *New England Journal of Medicine* 1985; 313(21): 1315–22. Interestingly, statistics indicate that human mortality from all causes is lowest at two A.M. and highest at eight A.M. *Encyclopedia of Sleep and Dreaming—1993* (New York: Macmillan Publishing Co., 1993).
5. American Heart Association. "Heart and Stroke Facts," 1995 Statistical Supplement.
6. Aoyama, H., Mori, N., and Mori, W. "Effects of Melatonin on Genetic Hypercholesterolemia in Rats." *Atherosclerosis* 1988; 69: 269–72.
7. Mori, N., Aoyama, H., and Mori, W. "Anti-Hypercholesterolemic Effect of Melatonin in Rats." *Japanese Society of Pathology* 1989; 39: 613–18.

8. Mori, W., Aoyama, H., and Mori, N. "Melatonin Protects Rats from Injurious Effects of Glucocorticoid, Dexamethasone." *Japanese Journal of Experimental Medicine* 1984; 54(6): 255–61.

9. Aoyama, H., Mori, N., and Mori, W. "Effects of Melatonin on Genetic Hypercholesterolemia in Rats." *Atherosclerosis* 1988; 69: 269–72.

10. Pierpaoli, W., Dall'ara, A., and Regelson, W. "The Pineal Control of Aging: The Effects of Melatonin and Pineal Grafting on the Survival of Older Mice." *Annals of the New York Academy of Sciences* 1991; 621:291–313.

11. Muller-Wieland, D., Behnke, B., and Krone, W. "Melatonin Inhibits LDL Receptor Activity and Cholesterol Synthesis in Freshly Isolated Human Mononuclear Leukocytes." *Biochemical and Biophysical Research Communications* 1994; 203(1): 416–21. They mention the relationship between high cholesterol and low melatonin in this paper, but they have yet to publish their data supporting this observation.

12. Muller-Wieland, D., Behnke, B., and Krone, W. "Melatonin Inhibits LDL Receptor Activity and Cholesterol Synthesis in Freshly Isolated Human Mononuclear Leukocytes." *Biochemical and Biophysical Research Communications* 1994; 203(1): 416–21.

13. Cohen M., Josimovich J., and Brzezinksi A. *Melatonin From Contraception to Breast Cancer Prevention* (Maryland: Sheba Press, 1995).

14. Angier, N. "Health Benefits from Soy Protein." *New York Times*, Aug. 3, 1995, p. A1.

15. Long, J.W., and Rybacki, J.J. *The Essential Guide to Prescription Drugs—1995* (New York: HarperPerennial, 1995).

16. Chapman, V. "Is Lipoprotein Oxidation Crucial for Heart Disease Process?" *University Week* 1994 Jan. 6

17. Hodis, H.N., et al. *Journal of the American Medical Association* 1995; 273(23): 1849–54.

18. Pieri, C., Marra, M., Moroni, F., and Marcheselli, F.

"Melatonin: A Peroxyl Radical Scavenger More Effective than Vitamin E." *Pergamon* 1994; 55(15): 271–76.

19. Brugger. P., Marktl, W., and Herold, M. "Impaired Nocturnal Secretion of Melatonin in Coronary Heart Disease." *Lancet* 1995 June 3; 345: 1408.

20. In their paper cited in note 19, Brugger et al. present a new theory by which melatonin might help prevent heart disease. They noted that at night concentrations of urinary norepinephrine (noradrenaline) are higher in patients with coronary heart disease than in healthy patients. Melatonin significantly reduces norepinephrine turnover in the heart. Elevated norepinephrine may be involved in the damage to the artery vessel wall, "because the atherogenic uptake of low-density-lipoprotein cholesterol is accelerated by these amines at pathophysiological concentrations." Further evidence that supports this theory was published in 1980 in a paper by Cunnane et al. showing pinealectomized rats had increased vascular reactivity to vasoconstrictor agents, including norepinephrine. See Cunnane, S.C., Manku, M.S., and Horrobin, D.F. "Enhanced Vascular Reactivity to Various Vasoconstrictor Agents Following Pinealectomy in the Rat: Role of Melatonin." *Cancer Journal of Physiology and Pharmacology* 1980; 58: 287–93.

21. Statistics are from the American Heart Association publication "Heart and Stroke Facts," 1995 Statistical Supplement.

22. Holmes, S.W., and Sugden, D. "The Effect of Melatonin on Pinealectomy-induced Hypertension in the Rat." *Proceedings of the B.P.S.* 1975 Dec.: 306.

23. Kawashima, K., Nagakura, A., and Spector, S. "Melatonin in Serum and the Pineal of Spontaneously Hypertensive Rats." *Clincal and Experimental Hypertension—Theory and Practice* 1984; A6(8): 1517–28.

24. Birau, N. *Melatonin in Human Serum: Progress in Screening Investigation and Clinic* (Institute of Preven-

tive Endocrinology, Bremen, Federal Republic of Germany, 1980).

25. Brismar, K., Hylander, B., and Wetterberg, L. "Melatonin Secretion Related to Side-effects of B-Blockers from the Central Nervous System." *Acta Medica Scandinavica* 1988; 223: 525–30.

26. Note: One milligram of melatonin was administered to each nostril.

27. Birau, N., Peterssen, U., and Gottschalk, J. "Hypotensive Effect of Melatonin in Essential Hypertension." *IRCS Medical Science* 1981; 9: 906.

28. Cohen, M., Josimovich, J., and Brzezinski, A. *Melatonin: From Contraception to Breast Cancer Prevention* (Potomac, Maryland: Sheba Press, 1995), p. 76.

29. Ceriello, A., Guigliano, D., and Lefebvre, P.J. "Anti-Oxidants Show an Anti-Hypertensive Effect in Diabetic and Hypertensive Subjects." *Clinical Science* 1991; 81: 739–42.

30. Weekley, L.B. "Melatonin-Induced Relaxation of Rat Aorta: Interaction with Adrenergic Agonists." *Journal of Pineal Research* 1991; 11: 28–34.

31. "Blood-Pressure Drugs Gain," *New York Times*, April 25, 1995, p. B10.

32. "Blood-Pressure Drugs Gain," *New York Times*, April 25, 1995, p. B10.

33. Vacas, M., Del Zar, M., and Cardinali, D. "Inhibition of Human Platelet Aggregation and Thromboxane B_2 Production by Melatonin. Correlation with Plasma Melatonin Levels." *Munksgaard* 1991: 135–39.

34. Flitter, W.D. "Free Radicals and Myocardial Reperfusion Injury." *British Medical Bulletin* 1993; 49(3): 545–55.

35. Weitz, Z.W., Birnbaum, A.J., and Skosey, J.L. "High Breath Pentane Concentrations During Acute Myocardial Infarction." *Lancet* 1991; 337: 933–35.

36. Blatt, C.M., Rabinowitz, S.H., and Lown, B. "Central Serotonergic Agents Raise the Repetitive Extrasystole Threshold of the Vulnerable Period of the Canine

Ventricular Myocardium." *Circulation Research* 1979; 44(5): 723–30.

CHAPTER 8: UNLOCKING THE SLEEP GATE

1. Dollins, A.B., Wurtman, R.J., and Deng, M.H. "Effect of Inducing Nocturnal Serum Melatonin Concentrations in Daytime on Sleep, Mood, Body Temperature, and Performance." *Proceedings of the National Academy of Sciences* 1994; 91: 1824–28. The study was not published until 1994, but preliminary results were announced in 1993.
2. For a review of melatonin sleep research, see Dawson, D., and Encel, N. "Melatonin and Sleep in Humans," *Journal of Pineal Research* 1993; 15: 1–12.
3. "Wake Up America: A National Sleep Alert," Executive Summary and Volume One Overview of the Report of the National Commission on Sleep Disorders Research. Submitted to the United States Congress. DHHS Pub. No. 92-XXXX (Washington, DC; Sup., 1992).
4. *Encyclopedia of Sleep and Dreaming* (New York: Macmillan Publishing Co., 1993), p. 703. (Carskadon, MA, ed., p. 426.)
5. *Encyclopedia of Sleep and Dreaming* (New York: Macmillan Publishing Co., 1993), p. 703. (Carskadon, MA, ed., p. 73–74.)
6. Kales, A. "Benzodiazepine Hypnotics and Insomnia." *Hospital Practice* 1990; 25 (Suppl 3): 7–21.
7. *Encyclopedia of Sleep and Dreaming* (New York: Macmillan Publishing Co., 1993), p. 703. (Carskadon, MA, ed., p. 73.)
8. *Encyclopedia of Sleep and Dreaming* (New York: Macmillan Publishing Co., 1993), p. 703. (Carskadon, MA, ed., p. 563.)
9. Greenblatt, D.J. "Pharmacology of Benzodiazepine

Hypnotics." *Journal of Clinical Psychiatry* 1992; 53(Suppl 6): 7–13.

10. There is evidence that elements of the immune system, in particular the cytokine IL-1, can induce sleep. This might be a melatonin-mediated event. IL-1 increases heat production in the body, and it has been shown that raising the body temperature enhances production of melatonin. *Encyclopedia of Sleep and Dreaming* (New York: Macmillan Publishing Co., 1993), p. 295.

11. The air force has sponsored numerous studies on the virtues of napping because on some occasions pilots must fly long missions and do not have the opportunity to get a full eight hours' rest. To keep their pilots combat ready, they have trained them to relinquish the controls and take thirty-minute "power naps," which keep them fairly rested without feeling groggy. If they must take longer naps, they are advised to nap for three or more hours so they will have sufficient time to cycle in and out of slow wave sleep.

12. Steinberg, R., and Soyka, M. "Problems in Long-Term Benzodiazepine Treatment." *Schweizerische Rundschau für Medizin Praxis* 1989; 78: 784–87.

13. Shorr, R.I., et al. "Failure to Limit Quantities of Benzodiazepine Hypnotic Drugs for Outpatients: Placing the Elderly at Risk." *American Journal of Medicine* 1990; 89(6): 725–32.

14. Cramer, H., Rudolph, J., and Kendel, K. "On the Effects of Melatonin on Sleep and Behavior in Man." *Advances in Biochemical Psychopharmacology* 1974; 11: 187–91.

15. This was a placebo-controlled, double-blind, crossover study.

16. Rod Hughes, personal communication. This study was published in *Sleep Research* in 1994.

17. Singer, C., Wild, K., Sack, R., and Lewy, A. "High Dose Melatonin Is Well Tolerated by the Elderly." *Sleep Research* 1994; 23: 86.

18. Data not yet published.

19. Rod Hughes, personal communication.

20. Rod Hughes, personal communication.

21. Lieberman, H.R., Waldhauser, F., and Wurtman, R.J. "Effects of Melatonin on Human Mood and Performance." *Brain Research* 1984; 323: 201–07.

22. Zhdanova, I.V., Wurtman, R.J., and Schomer, D.L. "Sleep-inducing Effects of Low Doses of Melatonin Ingested in the Evening." *Clinical Pharmacology and Therapeutics* 1995; 57: 552–58.

23. Lakshmi Putcha, personal communication. Medical Science Division, Johnson Space Center, Houston, TX.

24. The need for a program to help remedy the sleep problems of astronauts was reported in an article in the *Clinical Investigator* 1993; 71(9): 718–24.

25. To buttress the argument that melatonin influences sleep directly, some researchers point to the fact that it functions very much like traditional sleep aids, in that higher amounts appear to have a greater sleep-inducing effect than smaller amounts. In a study submitted for publication, Rod Hughes, a researcher now at OHSU, and Jon French at Brooks Air Force Base conducted a study comparing 10-milligram and 100-milligram doses of melatonin and found a marked dose-dependent effect on both body temperature and sleepiness.

26. Campbell, S.S., and Broughton, R.J. "Rapid Decline in Body Temperature Before Sleep: Fluffing the Physiological Pillow?" *Chronobiology International* April 1994; 11(2): 126–31.

27. Horne, J. A., and Shackell, B.S. "Slow Wave Sleep Elevations After Body Heating: Proximity to Sleep and Effects of Aspirin." *Sleep* 1987; 10(4): 383–92. I wonder if being in a warm room also raises one's melatonin levels, which could explain why this environment is so soporific.

    Interestingly, taking a hot bath at night also increases the proportion of time you spend in slow wave sleep. This sleep-deepening effect could be caused by melatonin. One indication that it could is that taking an aspirin along with a hot bath prevents you from sleeping more deeply. As we will see in Chapter 15, aspirin inhibits production of melatonin.

Another insight to come from this and other studies is that pineal gland may play an important role in regulating body temperature, producing higher levels of melatonin as a person's temperature rises. The increased levels of melatonin would have a temperature-lowering effect. Researcher Patricia Murphy is now exploring melatonin's potential as an antipyretic or fever reducer. It would be the first fever medication that would simultaneously lower body temperature and stimulate the immune system, helping to relieve discomfort and speed healing as well.

28. Hughes, R.J., Sack, R.L., Singer, C.M., and Lewy, A.J. "A Comparison of the Hypnotic Efficacy of Melatonin and Temazepam on Nocturnal Sleep in Healthy Adults." *Sleep Research*.

29. Hagan, R.M., and Oakley, N.R. "Melatonin Comes of Age?" *Trends in Pharmacological Sciences* 1995; 16: 81–83.

30. Campbell, S.S., Gillin, J.C., Kripke, D.F., and Clopton, P. "Gender Differences in the Circadian Temperature Rhythms of Healthy Elderly Subjects: Relationships to Sleep Quality." *Sleep* 1989; 12(6): 529–36.

31. Copinschi, G., and Van Cauter, E. "Effects of Ageing on Modulation of Hormonal Secretions by Sleep and Circadian Rhythmicity." *Hormone Research* 1995; 43: 20–24.

32. Haimov, I., Laudon, M., Zisapel, M., Surjon, M., Nof, D., Schlitner, A., and Lavie, P. "The Relationship Between Urinary 6-Sulphatoxymelatonin Rhythm and Insomnia in Old Age." In *Advances in Pineal Research* vol. 8, ed. M. Møller and P. Pévet (London: John Libbey and Co., 1994), pp. 433–38.

The investigators measured a metabolite of melatonin, 6-sulphatoxymelatonin, in the urine, which corresponds very closely with serum melatonin levels. The group that did not sleep well had 1.9 +/ − .9 μg/h and the good sleepers had 3.3 +/− 2.1 μg/h (P < 0.01).

33. Cliff Singer, personal communication.

34. Rod Hughes, personal communication.

35. The timing of the administration of the melatonin was adjusted to match each person's biological rhythms.

36. Stankov, B., Fraschini, F., and Oldani, A. "Melatonin and Delayed Sleep Phase Syndrome: Ambulatory Polygraphic Evaluation." *NeuroReport* 1994; 6: 132–34.

CHAPTER 9: BACK IN SYNC

1. The SCN is so small that researchers discovered it in humans only about a decade ago.

2. We owe this insight to a large extent to Alfred J. Lewy, from the Oregon Health Sciences University. He was able to show that melatonin is the most accurate marker of the output of the body clock, giving chronobiologists their most reliable tool for determining what "time" it is in the body.

3. The technical name for the pineal gland is *neuroendocrine transducer*, which means that it translates information from the nervous system into a hormone.

4. According to the time that you administer melatonin, you can advance or delay the body clock. Robert Sack and Alfred Lewy have worked out the "phase-response curve," or PRC, of melatonin therapy with great accuracy. For a good article summarizing the information, see Lewy, A.J., Ahmed, S., and Sack, R.L.

"Melatonin Shifts Human Circadian Rhythms According to a Phase-Response Curve." *Chronobiology International* 1992; 9(5): 380–92.

5. Melbin, M. *Night as Frontier: Colonizing the World After Dark* (New York: Free Press, 1987), p. 27.

6. Wright, K.P., Badia, P., Myers, B.L., and Hakel, M. "Effects of Caffeine, Bright Light, and Their Combination on Nighttime Melatonin and Temperature During Two Nights of Sleep Deprivation." *Sleep Research* 1995; 24: 458.

7. Arendt, J. "Human Responses to Light and Melatonin." In *Advances in Pineal Research*, vol. 8, ed. M. Møller and P. Pévet (London: John Libbey and Co., 1994), pp. 439–41.

8. Arendt, J., et al. "Alleviation of Jet Lag by Melatonin: Preliminary Results of Controlled Double Blind Trial." *British Medical Journal* 1986; 292: 1170.

9. Lino, A., Silvy, S., and Rusconi, A. "Melatonin and Jet Lag: Treatment Schedule." *Biological Psychiatry* 1993; 34: 587–88.

10. Claustrat, B., Brun, J., and Chazot, G. "Melatonin and Jet Lag: Confirmatory Result Using a Simplified Protocol." *Biological Psychiatry* 1992; 32: 705–11.

11. Peggy Whitson, personal communication.

12. Neville, K.J., French, J., and Storm, W.F. "Subjective Fatigue of C-141 Aircrews During Operation Desert Storm." *Human Factors* 1994; 36(2): 339–49.

CHAPTER 10: A MASTER SEX HORMONE

1. Later, Hoffman and I showed that female ovaries also respond to seasonal signals from the pineal gland.

2. "Seasonal Variation of Twin Births in Washington State." *Acta Geneticae Medicae et Gemellologiae* 1993; 42: 141–9.

3. Rojansky, N., Brzezinski, A., and Schenker, J.G.

"Seasonality in Human Reproduction: An Update." *Human Reproduction* 1992; 7: 735–45.

4. Cook, F.A. "Medical Observations Among the Esquimaux." *Transactions of the New York Obstetrical Society* 1894; 3: 282–91.

5. Bary Wilson, personal communication. Data not yet published.

6. Laughlin, G.A., Loucks, A.B., and Yen S.S.C. "Marked Augmentation of Nocturnal Melatonin Secretion in Amenorrheic Athletes, but Not in Cycling Athletes: Unaltered by Opioidergic or Dopaminergic Blockade." *Journal of Clinical Endocrinology and Metabolism* 1991; 73(6): 1321–26. High levels of melatonin could be due to the body's attempts to counter the free radicals produced during strenuous exercise.

7. Rookus, M.A. and Van Leeuwen, F.E. "Oral contraceptives and Risk of Breast Cancer in Women Aged 20–54 years." *Lancet* 1994; 344: 844–85. These researchers have found that "four or more years of oral contraceptive use, especially if before the age of 20, is associated with an increased risk of breast cancer developing at an early age."

8. Long, J.W., and Rybacki, J.J. *The Essential Guide to Prescription Drugs—1995* (New York: HarperPerennial, 1995).

9. Cohen, M., Josimovich, J., and Brzezinski, A. *Melatonin: From Contraception to Breast Cancer Prevention* (Potomac, Maryland: Sheba Press, 1995).

10. Parry, B.L., Berga, S.L., and Gillin, J.C. *Chronobiology: Its Role in Clinical Medicine, General Biology and Agriculture. Melatonin and Phototherapy in Premenstrual Depression* (Wiley-Liss, 1990), pp. 35–43.

11. Michael Cohen, personal communication. Cohen believes that melatonin alleviates the symptoms of PMS because it reduces the size of the follicles that are recruited during the menstrual cycle. It has been known for many years, he says, that anything that

reduces the size of the follicles has a positive effect on PMS.

12. Sarafina Corsella, personal communication.

13. Parry, B.L., Berga, S.L., and Gillin, J.C. *Chronobiology: Its Role in Clinical Medicine, General Biology and Agriculture. Melatonin and Phototherapy in Premenstrual Depression* (Wiley-Liss, 1990), pp. 35–43.

14. Sack, R.L., Lewy, A.J., and Singer, C.M. "Human Melatonin Production Decreases with Age." *Journal of Pineal Research* 1986; 3: 379–88.

15. Fernandez, B., Malde, J.L., and Acuna, D. "Relationship Between Adenohypophyseal and Steroid Hormones and Variations in Serum and Urinary Melatonin Levels During the Ovarian Cycle, Perimenopause, and Menopause in Healthy Women." *Steroid Biochemistry* 1990; 35(2): 257–62.

16. Kornhauser, C., et al. "High Prevalence of Arterial Hypertension in Women over 50 Years." *Revista de investigación clínica* 1994; 46(4): 287–94.

17. Ushiroyama, T., et al. "Plasma Lipid and Lipoprotein Levels in Perimenopausal Women." *Acta Obstetricia et Gynecologica Scandinavica* 1993; 72: 428–33.

18. Kannel, W.B., and Wilson P.W. "Risk Factors that Attenuate the Female Coronary Disease Advantage." *Archives of Internal Medicine* 1995; 155: 57–61.

19. Terzolo, M., Piovesan, A., and Angeli, A. "Effects of Long-Term, Low-Dose, Time-Specified Melatonin Administration on Endocrine and Cardiovascular Variables in Adult Men." *Journal of Pineal Research* 1990; 9: 113–24.

20. Oaknin-Bendahan, S., Anis, Y., and Zisapel, N. "Effects of Long-term Administration of Melatonin and a Putative Antagonist on the Ageing Rat." *NeuroReport* 1995; 6: 785–88.

21. Van Vuuren, R.J., Du Plessis, D.J., and Theron, J.J. "Melatonin in Human Semen." *South African Medical Journal* 1988; 73: 375–76. Melatonin may be influencing sperm motility by affecting the sliding mechanism of the microtubular complex in the flagellum.

CHAPTER 11: MELATONIN AND YOUR MIND

1. Reiter, R.J., and Vaughan, M.K. *Endocrinology: People and Ideas* (American Physiological Society, 1988), pp. 215–37.

2. Beck-Friis, J., Kjellman, B.F., and Wetterberg, L. "Serum Melatonin in Relation to Clinical Variables in Patients with Major Depressive Disorder and a Hypothesis of a Low Melatonin Syndrome." *Acta Psychiatrica Scandinavica* 1985; 71: 319–30. One type of depression linked with low melatonin is melancholia, a mood disorder characterized by an inability to experience pleasure, a decreased interest in food, and a worsening of mood in the morning. A second type, named "low melatonin syndrome depression," has the following characteristics: 1. Low nocturnal melatonin, 2. Abnormal dexamethasone suppression test, 3. Disturbed 24-h rhythm of cortisol, 4. Less pronounced daily and annual cyclic variation in depressive symptomatology.

3. Cavallo, A., Holt, K.G., and Meyer, W.J. "Melatonin Circadian Rhythm in Childhood Depression." *Journal of the American Academy of Child and Adolescent Psychiatry* 1987; 26(3): 395–99.

4. Beck-Friis, J., Kjellman, B.F., and Wetterberg, L. "Serum Melatonin in Relation to Clinical Variables in Patients with Major Depressive Disorder and a Hypothesis of a Low Melatonin Syndrome." *Acta Psychiatrica Scandinavica* 1985; 71: 319–30.

5. Goleman, D. "Severe Trauma May Damage the Brain as Well as the Psyche," *New York Times*, Aug. 1, 1995, p. B8.

6. Stanley, M., and Brown, G.M. "Melatonin Levels Are Reduced in the Pineal Glands of Suicide Victims." *Psychopharmacology* 1988; 24(3): 484–87.

7. Oxenkrug, G.F., McIntyre, I.M., and McCauley, R.B. "Single Dose of Tranylcypromine Increases Human Plasma Melatonin." *Biological Psychiatry* 1986; 21:1081–85.

8. Pang, S.F. "Abstracts of Free Communication." *Journal of Neural Transmission* 1986; Suppl 21:479–504. Researchers have suggested that lithium alters the amount of light that enters the eyes, which would explain why the drug influences melatonin production.

9. Chazot, G., Claustrat, B., and Olivier, M. "Rapid Antidepressant Activity of Destyr Gamma Endorphin: Correlation with Urinary Melatonin." *Biological Psychiatry* 1985; 20: 1026–30.

10. Souetre, E., Salvati, E., and Darcourt, G. "5-Methoxypsoralen Increases the Plasma Melatonin Levels in Humans." *Journal of Investigative Dermatology* 1987; 89: 152–55.

11. Huether, G., Hajak, G., Poeggeler, B., and Ruther, E. "The Metabolic Fate of infused L-Tryptophan in Men: Possible Clinical Implications of the Accumulation of Circulating Tryptophan and Trytophan Metabolites." *Psychopharmacology* 1992; 109: 422–32.

12. Levitt, A.J., Brown, G.M., and Stern, K.B. "Tryptophan Treatment and Melatonin Response in a Patient with Seasonal Affective Disorder." *Journal of Clinical Psychopharmacology* 1991; 11(1): 74–75.

13. Demisch, L. *Clinical Pharmacology of Melatonin Regulation.* (Boca Raton: CRC Press, 1993).

14. The subjects were injected with 1.25 milligrams of melatonin per kilogram of body weight.

15. Anton-Tay, F., "On the Effects of Melatonin upon Human Brain: Its Possible Therapeutic Implications." *Life Sciences* 1971; 10: 841–50.

16. Miles, A., and Philbrick, D.R.S. "Melatonin and Psychiatry." *Biological Psychiatry* 1988; 23: 405–25.

17. Arendt, J. "Melatonin: A New Probe in Psychiatric Investigation." *British Journal of Psychiatry* 1989; 155: 585–90.

18. Kennedy, S.H., Tighe, S., and Brown, G.M. "Melatonin and Cortisol 'Switches' During Mania, Depression, and Euthymia in a Drug-Free Bipolar Patient."

Journal of Nervous and Mental Disease 1989; 177(5): 300–03.

19. Claustrat, B., Brun, J., and Chazot, G. "Melatonin in Humans, Neuroendocrinological and Pharmacological Aspects." *Nuclear Medicine and Biology* 1990; 17(7): 625–32.

20. Monteleone, P., Maj, M., Fusco, M., Kemali, D., and Reiter, R.J. "Depressed Nocturnal Plasma Melatonin Levels in Drug-Free Paranoid Schizophrenics." *Schizophrenia Research* 1992; 7: 77–84. Note that this was not the first study to report on the melatonin levels of schizophrenics. But this one was designed to correct some of the weaknesses of the earlier studies. We included a control group, we measured melatonin levels at night, we made sure that the subjects were drug free, and we measured their melatonin production at seven different time periods during the night, rather than just one, as had been the case in some earlier studies.

21. Some of the similarities they noted were that pain sufferers and those with depression tend to have high concentrations of certain endorphins, low concentrations of a serotonin metabolite, low amounts of MAO in platelets, and abnormal dexamethasone suppression tests.

22. Almay, B.G.L., Von Knorring, L., and Wetterberg, L. "Melatonin in Serum and Urine in Patients with Idiopathic Pain Syndromes." *Psychiatry Research* 1987; 22: 179–91. The researchers in this study also observed a relationship between low melatonin levels and a variety of other complaints. People with a relative deficiency of the hormone had a greater incidence of sadness, inner tension, concentration difficulties, and memory disturbances.

23. Lakin, M.L., Miller, C.H., and Winters, W.D. "Involvement of the Pineal Gland and Melatonin in Murine Analgesia." *Life Sciences* 1981; 29: 2543–51.

24. Kavaliers, M., Hirst, M., and Teskey, G.C. "Ageing,

Opioid Analgesic and the Pineal Gland." *Life Sciences* 1983; 32: 2279–87.

25. Our maximum pain threshold coincides with our minimum body temperature, and body temperature is strongly correlated with melatonin levels.

26. Kolata, G., "Study Says 1 in 5 Americans Suffers from Chronic Pain," *New York Times*, Oct. 21, 1994, p. A1.

27. Wetterberg, L. "Melatonin in Humans: Physiological and Clinical Studies." *Journal of Neural Transmission* 1978; Suppl. 13: 289–310.

28. Wetterberg, L., Aperia, B., and Yuwiler, A. "Age, Alcoholism and Depression are Associated with Low Levels of Urinary Melatonin." *Journal of Psychiatry and Neuroscience* 1992; 17(5): 215–24.

29. Isabel Davidoff, director of D/ART, National Institute of Mental Health, letter to the editor, *New York Times*, Jan. 9, 1994.

30. Wurtman, R.J., and Wurtman, J.J. "Carbohydrates and Depression." *Scientific American* 1989 Jan.; 68–75.

31. Carskadon, M.A., and Acebo, C. "Parental Reports of Seasonal Mood and Behavior Changes in Children." *Journal of the American Academy of Child and Adolescent Psychiatry* 1993; 32(2): 246.

32. Wehr, T.A. "The Durations of Human Melatonin Secretion and Sleep Respond to the Changes in Daylength (Photoperiod)." *Journal of Clinical Endocrinology and Metabolism* 1991; 73(6): 1276–80.

33. Wehr, T.A. "The Durations of Human Melatonin Secretion and Sleep Respond to the Changes in Daylength (Photoperiod)." *Journal of Clinical Endocrinology and Metabolism* 1991; 73(6): 1276–80. Other studies looking at sleeping habits of people in their everyday situations have shown that people sleep more in the winter the farther north or south they are from the equator.

34. Krauchi, K., Wirz-Justice, A., and Graw, P. "The Relationship of Affective Disorder State to Dietary Preference: Winter Depression and Light Therapy as a Model." *Journal of Affective Disorders* 1990; 20: 43–53.

35. Rao, M.L., Muller-Oerlinghausen, B., and Volz, H.P. "The Influence of Phototherapy on Serotonin and Melatonin in Non-seasonal Depression." *Pharmacopsychiatry* 1990; 23: 155–58.
36. Blundell, J.E. "Serotonin and Appetite." *Neuropharmacology* 1984; 23(128): 1537–51.
37. Lewy, A.J., Kern, H.A., Rosenthal, N.E., and Wehr, T.A. "Bright Artificial Light Treatment of a Manic-Depressive Patient with a Seasonal Mood Cycle." *American Journal of Psychiatry* 1982; 139(11): 1496–98.

CHAPTER 12: THE GREAT ANTI-AGING EXPERIMENT

1. As long ago as the late 1950s, evidence suggested an association between the pineal gland and longevity. During the subsequent years, evidence supporting this contention has accumulated intermittently. But this experiment was the first placebo-controlled study that relied on melatonin supplementation.
2. Maestroni, G.J., Conti, A., and Pierpaoli, W. "Pineal Melatonin, Its Fundamental Immunoregulatory Role in Aging and Cancer." *Annals of the New York Academy of Sciences* 1988; 521: 140–48.
3. Free radicals may even play a role in our decreasing production of melatonin. The part of the brain that sends the signal to the pineal gland to produce melatonin, the SCN, becomes damaged over time by a brain chemical called glutamate, which causes the formation of a variety of toxic radicals. As the neurons in the SCN become increasingly damaged, they send out a weaker and more erratic signal.
4. Harman, D. "Free Radical Theory of Aging." *Mutation Research* 1992; 275: 257–66.
5. Yu, B.P. *Free Radicals in Aging* (Boca Raton: CRC Press, 1993), p. 301.

6. Reiter, R.J. "The Pineal Gland and Melatonin in Relation to Aging: A Summary of the Theories and of the Data." *Experimental Gerontology* 1995; 30: 199–212. Also, "Oxidative Processes and Antioxidative Defense Mechanisms in the Aging Brain." *FASEB Journal* 1995; 9: 526–33.

7. All of the surviving rats were sacrificed at 27 to 29 months of age, so there was no opportunity to observe how much longer they might live.

8. Oaknin-Bendahan, S., Anis, Y., and Zisapel, N. "Effects of Long-term Administration of Melatonin and a Putative Antagonist on the Ageing Rat." *NeuroReport* 1995; 6: 785–88.

9. Stokkan, K.-A., Reiter, R.J., and Vaughan, M.K. "Food Restriction Retards Aging of the Pineal Gland." *Brain Research* 1991; 545: 66–72.

10. Walker, R.F., McMahon, K.M., and Pivorun, E.B. "Pineal Gland Structure and Respiration as Affected by Age and Hypocaloric Diet." *Experimental Gerontology* 1978; 13: 91–99.

11. Magnani, M., and Accorsi, A. "The Female Longevity Phenomenon. Hypothesis on Some Molecular and Cell Biology Aspects." *Mechanisms of Ageing and Development* 1993; 72: 89–95.

12. Touitou, Y., Fevre-Montange, M., and Nakache, J.P. "Age and Sex-Associated Modification of Plasma Melatonin Concentrations in Man. Relationship to Pathology, Malignant or Not, and Autopsy Findings." *Acta Endocrinologica* 1985; 108: 135–44.

13. Almay, B.G.L., Von Knorring, L., and Wetterberg, L. "Melatonin in Serum and Urine in Patients with Idiopathic Pain Syndromes." *Psychiatry Research* 1987; 22: 179–91.

14. Birau, N. *Melatonin in Human Serum: Progress in Screening Investigation and Clinic* (Institute of Preventive Endocrinology, Bremen, Federal Republic of Germany, 1980).

15. Beal, M.F. "Energy, Oxidative Damage, and Alzheimer's Disease: Clues to the Underlying Puzzle."

Neurobiology of Aging 1994; 15 (Suppl 2): 171–74.

16. Kolata, G. "Brain Scans May Foretell Alzheimer's," *New York Times*, Mar. 24, 1995, p. A11.

17. Murialdo, G., Castelli, P., and Dolleri, A. "Circadian Secretion of Melatonin and Thyrotropin in Hospitalized Aged Patients." 1993 Feb. 5(1): 39–46. *Aging Clinical and Experimental Research*.

18. Mishima, K., Okawa, M., and Takahashi, K. "Morning Bright Light Therapy for Sleep and Behavior Disorders in Elderly Patients with Dementia." *Acta Psychiatrica Scandinavica* 1994; 89: 1–7.

19. Reiter. R.J., Poeggeler, B., Chen, L-D., and Barlow-Walden, L.R. "Melatonin as a Free Radical Scavenger: Theoretical Implications for Neurodegenerative Disorders in the Aged." Unpublished.

20. Sansoni, P., Brianti, V., and Franceshi, C. "NK Cell Activity and T-Lymphocyte Proliferation in Healthy Centenarians." *Annals of the New York Academy of Sciences* 1992; 663: 505–07.

21. Smythe, G.A., Lazarus, L. "Growth Hormone Response to Melatonin in Man." *Science* 1974; 184: 1373.

22. Valcavi, R., Zini, M., Maestroni, G.J., and Conti, A. "Melatonin Stimulates Growth Hormone Secretion Through Pathways Other Than the Growth Hormone-Releasing Hormone." *Clinical Endocrinology* 1993; 39: 193–99.

CHAPTER 13: LET THERE BE LIGHT— AND DARK

1. Laakso, M-L., Porkka-Heiskanen, T., and Johansson, G. "Twenty-Four-Hour Patterns of Pineal Melatonin and Pituitary and Plasma Prolactin in Male Rats under 'Natural' and Artificial Lighting Conditions." *Neuroendocrinology* 1988; 48: 308–13.

2. Espiritu, R.C., Kripke, D.F., and Kaplan, O.J. "Low Illumination Experienced by San Diego Adults: Association with Atypical Depressive Symptoms." *Biological Psychiatry* 1994; 35: 403–07.

3. Koller, M., Kundi, M., Stidl, H-G., Zidek, T., and Haider, M. "Personal Light Dosimetry in Permanent Night and Day Workers." *Chronobiology International* 1993; 10: 143–55.

4. Personal communication.

5. McIntyre, I.M., Norman, T.R., and Burrows, G.D. "Melatonin Supersensitivity to Dim Light in Seasonal Affective Disorder." *Lancet* 1990; 335: 488.

6. Rao, M.L., Muller-Oerlinghausen, B., and Volz, H.P. "The Influence of Phototherapy on Serotonin and Melatonin in Non-seasonal Depression." *Pharmacopsychiatry* 1990; 23: 155–58.

7. Hansen, T., Bratlid, T., and Brenn, T. "Midwinter Insomnia in the Subarctic Region: Evening Levels of Serum Melatonin and Cortisol Before and After Treatment with Bright Artificial Light." *Acta Psychiatrica Scandinavica* 1987; 75: 428–34.

8. Grunberger, J., Linzmayer, L., and Saletu, B. "The Effect of Biologically-Active Light on the Noo- and Thymopsyche and on Psychophysiological Variables in Healthy Volunteers." *International Journal of Psychophysiology* 1993; 15: 27–37.

9. Rao, M.L., Muller-Oerlinghausen, B., and Volz, H.P. "Blood Serotonin, Serum Melatonin and Light Therapy in Healthy Subjects and in Patients with Non-seasonal Depression." *Acta Psychiatrica Scandinavica* 1992; 86: 127–32.

10. Espiritu, R.C., Kripke, D.F., Kaplan, O.J. "Low Illumination Experienced by San Diego Adults: Association with Atypical Depressive Symptoms." *Biological Psychiatry* 1994; 35: 403–07.

11. Reid, D.P. *The Tao of Health, Sex and Longevity.* (New York: Simon & Schuster, 1989), p. 247.

12. For an interesting exposition of the relationship be-

tween yoga, the pineal gland, and seasonal affective disorder or SAD, see E. Leskowitz, "Seasonal Affective Disorder and the Yoga Paradigm: A Reconsideration of the Pineal Gland," *Medical Hypothesis* 1990; 33: 155–58.

13. Lewy, A.J., Wehr, T.A., and Goodwin, F.K. "Light Suppresses Melatonin Secretion in Humans." *Science* 1980 Dec.; 210.

14. Murphy, D.G.M., Murphy, D.M., Palazidou, E., and Arendt, J. "Seasonal Affective Disorder: Response to Light as Measured by Electroencephalogram, Melatonin Suppression, and Cerebral Blood Flow." *British Journal of Psychiatry* 1993; 163: 327–31.

15. Charles Graham, personal communication.

16. Yamazaki, J., Sugishita, M., and Takahashi, K. "The Effects of Vitamin B12 on the Suppression of Melatonin Secretion Under Illumination." *Japanese Journal of Psychiatry and Neurology* 1991; 45(1): 169–72.

17. Byerley, W-F., et al. "Biological Effect of Bright Light." *Progress in Neuro-Psychopharmacology and Biological Psychiatry* 1989; 13(5): 683–86.

18. *Report of the National Commission on Sleep Disorders Research.* DHHS Pub. No. 92-XXXX (Washington, DC, 1992).

19. Irwin, M., et al. "Partial Sleep Deprivation Reduces Natural Killer Cell Activity in Humans." *Psychosomatic Medicine* 1994; 56(6): 493–98.

20. Espiritu, R.C., Kripke, D.F., and Kaplan, O.J. "Low Illumination Experienced by San Diego Adults: Association with Atypical Depressive Symptoms." *Biological Psychiatry* 1994; 35: 403–07.

21. Danziger, L. "Read It and Sleep." *Allure*, Oct. 1994, pp. 110–12.

CHAPTER 14: THE ELUSIVE ENEMY— ELECTROMAGNETIC FIELDS

1. Another name for an EMF of this nature is ELF, or extremely low frequency electromagnetic fields.
2. Wilson, B.W., Wright, C., and Anderson, L.E. "Evidence for an Effect of ELF Electromagnetic Fields on Human Pineal Gland Function." *Journal of Pineal Research* 1990; 9: 259–69. A second study demonstrating a link between electric blanket use and lowered melatonin levels has yet to be published. Maestroni, G.J., Conti, A., and Reiter, R., ed. *Advances in Pineal Research*, vol. 7. (London: John Libbey and Co., 1994), p. 306.
3. The Germans call migratory restlessness "Zugunruhe," a wonderfully evocative term.
4. Semm, P., Schneider, T., and Vollrath, L. "Effects of an Earth-Strength Magnetic Field on Electrical Activity of Pineal Cells." *Nature* 1980; 288: 607–08.
5. Wilson, B.W., Stevens, R.G., and Anderson, L.E. "Neuroendocrine Mediated Effects of Electromagnetic-Field Exposure: Possible Role of the Pineal Gland." *Life Sciences* 1989; 45: 1319–32.
6. Dubbels, R., Klenke, E., Manz, B., Terwey, J., and Schloot, W. "Melatonin Determination with a Newly Developed ELISA System. Interindividual Differences in the Response of the Human Pineal Gland to Magnetic Fields." *Advances in Pineal Research*, vol. 7, ed. G.J. Maestroni, A. Conti, and R.J. Reiter (London: John Libbey and Co., 1994), pp. 27–33.
7. "Correlation Between Heart Attacks and Magnetic Activity." *Nature* 277: 646–48.
8. Kay, R.W. "Geomagnetic Storms: Association with Incidence of Depression as Measured by Hospital Admission." *British Journal of Psychiatry* 1994 Mar.; 164(3): 403–09.
9. Bary Wilson, personal communication. Unpublished study.

10. Perry, T.S. "A Rational View of EMF." EMF and Health Magazine 1994; 94.

11. Baum, A., Mevissen, M., and Loscher, W. "A Histopathological Study on Alterations in DMBA-induced Mammary Carcinogenesis in Rats with 50 Hz, 100 uT Magnetic Field Exposure." Carcinogenesis 1995; 16(1): 119–25.

12. Baum, A., Mevissen, M., and Loscher, W. "A Histopathological Study on Alterations in DMBA-induced Mammary Carcinogenesis in Rats with 50 Hz, 100 uT Magnetic Field Exposure." Carcinogenesis 1995; 16(1): 119–25.

13. Bennett, W.R., Jr. "Power Lines Are Homely, Not Hazardous." Wall Street Journal, Aug. 10, 1994.

14. One note of assurance, however, is that Liburdy discovered in his test-tube experiments that EMF exposure less than 2mG did not interfere with melatonin's anticancer ability, giving some experimental data to support this cutoff point.

15. Wilson, B.W., Wright, C., and Anderson, L.E. "Evidence for an Effect of ELF Electromagnetic Fields on Human Pineal Gland Function." Journal of Pineal Research 1990; 9: 259–69. A second study demonstrating a link between electric blanket use and lowered melatonin levels has yet to be published.

16. Prata, S. EMF Handbook (Corte Madera, CA: Waite Group Press, 1993), pp. 62–63.

CHAPTER 15: DRUGS THAT DEPLETE MELATONIN

1. Murphy, P.J., Badia, P., Myers, B.L., and Wright, K.P., Jr. "Nonsteroidal Anti-Inflammatory Drugs Affect Normal Sleep Patterns in Humans." Physiology and Behavior 1994; 55(6): 1063–66.

2. NSAIDs block the synthesis of fatty acids called prostaglandins, which, in test-tube experiments, reduce

the ability of pineal cells to produce melatonin. Daniel Cardinali, M.D., Ph.D., of the University of Buenos Aires, has studied this process in detail. Cardinali, D.P., Ritta, M.N., and Pereyra, E. "Role of Prostaglandins in Rat Pineal Neuroeffector Junction. Changes in Melatonin and Norepinephrine Release in Vitro." *Endocrinology* 1982; 111(2): 530–34.

3. Surrall, K., Smith, J.A., and Padwick, D.J. "Effect of Ibuprofen and Indomethacin on Human Plasma Melatonin." *Journal of Pharmacy and Pharmacology* 1987; 39: 840–43.

4. Interestingly, melatonin and indomethacin are very similar in molecular structure. Melatonin, like indomethacin, is a potent inhibitor of prostaglandin synthesis. Also, indomethacin may have anticancer properties.

5. Murphy, P.J., Badia, P., Myers, B.L., and Wright, K.P., Jr. "Nonsteroidal Anti-Inflammatory Drugs Affect Normal Sleep Patterns in Humans." *Physiology and Behavior* 1994; 55(6): 1063–66.

6. Johnson, A.G, Nguyen, T.V., and Day, R.O. "Do Nonsteroidal Anti-Inflammatory Drugs Affect Blood Pressure?" *Annals of Internal Medicine* 1994 Aug. 15; 12(4): 289–300.

7. Bryan Myers, personal communication.

8. Long, J.W., and Rybacki, J.J. *The Essential Guide to Prescription Drugs—1995* (New York: HarperPerennial, 1995), p. 863.

9. Brismar, K., Hylander, B., and Wetterberg, L. "Melatonin Secretion Related to Side-effects of B-Blockers from the Central Nervous System." *Acta Medica Scandinavica* 1988; 223: 525–30.

10. Lithell, H., Haglund, K., and Ostman, J. "Are Effects of Antihypertensive Treatment on Lipoproteins Merely 'Side-effects'?" *Acta Medica Scandinavica* 1988; 223: 531–36.

11. Muller-Wieland, D., Behnke, B., and Krone, W. "Melatonin Inhibits LDL Receptor Activity and Cholesterol Synthesis in Freshly Isolated Human

Mononuclear Leukocytes." *Biochemical and Biophysical Research Communications* 1994; 203(1): 416–21.

12. Long, J.W., and Rybacki, J.J. *The Essential Guide to Prescription Drugs-1995* (New York: HarperPerennial, 1995), p. 1064.

13. Meyer, A.C., Nieuwenhuis, J.J., and Meyer, B.J. "Dihydropyridine Calcium Antagonists Depress the Amplitude of the Plasma Melatonin Cycle in Baboons." *Life Sciences* 1986; 39: 1563–69.

14. Umeda, T., Naomi, S., Sato, T., et al. "Timing for Administration of an Antihypertensive Drug in the Treatment of Essential Hypertension." *Hypertension* 1994 Jan. 23; (1 Suppl): I 211–14.

15. Lewy, A.J., Siever, L.J., and Markey, S.P. "Clonidine Reduces Plasma Melatonin Levels." *Journal of Pharmacy and Pharmacology* 1986; 38: 555–56.

16. Not to be confused with Zantac, a drug prescribed for stomach problems.

17. McIntyre, I., Burrows, G.D., and Norman, T.R. "Suppression of Plasma Melatonin by a Single Dose of the Benzodiazepine Alprozolam in Humans." *Biological Psychiatry* 1988; 24: 105–08; Monteleone, P., Forziati, D., and Maj, M. "Preliminary Observations on the Suppression of Nocturnal Plasma Melatonin Levels by Short-Term Administraton of Diazepam in Humans." *Journal of Pineal Research* 1989; 6: 253–58.

18. McIntyre, I., Burrows, G.D., and Norman, T.R. "Suppression of Plasma Melatonin by a Single Dose of the Benzodiazepine Alprozolam in Humans." *Biological Psychiatry* 1988; 24: 105–08.

19. Hubain, P.P., et al. "Alprazolam and Amitriptyline in the Treatment of Major Depressive Disorder: A Double-Blind Clinical and Sleep EEG Study." *Journal of Affective Disorders*, 1990 Jan.; 18(1): 67–73.

20. Not yet available for sale in the United States.

21. Childs, P.A., Rodin, I., and Thompson, C. "Effect of Fluoxetine on Melatonin in Patients with Seasonal Affective Disorder and Matched Controls." *British Journal of Psychiatry* 1995; 166: 196–98.

22. Long, J.W., and Rybacki, J.J. *The Essential Guide to Prescription Drugs—1995* (New York: HarperPerennial).

23. Honma, K., Kohsaka, M., and Honma, S. "Effects of Vitamin B12 on Plasma Melatonin Rhythm in Humans: Increased Light Sensitivity Phase-Advances the Circadian Clock." *Experientia* 1992; 48: 716–20.

24. Wright, K.P., Badia, P., Myers, B.L., and Hakel, M. "Effects of Caffeine, Bright Light, and Their Combination on Nighttime Melatonin and Temperature During Two Nights of Sleep Deprivation." *Sleep Research* 1995; 24: 458. The authors suggest that caffeine intereferes with melatonin production by blocking the action of adenosine, a neuromodulator.

25. Wright, Jr., K.P., Badia, P., and Hakel, M. "The Combined Effects of Bright Light and Caffeine on Nighttime Alertness and Performance During Two Nights of Sleep Deprivation." *Sleep Research* 1995; 24: 459.

26. Wright, K.P., Badia, P., Myers, B.L., and Hakel, M. "Effects of Caffeine, Bright Light, and Their Combination on Nighttime Melatonin and Temperature During Two Nights of Sleep Deprivation. *Sleep Research* 1995; 24: 460.

27. *Encyclopedia of Sleep and Dreaming.* (New York: Macmillan Publishing Co., 1993), p. 703.

28. Lindsted, K.D., et al. "Coffee Consumption and Cause-Specific Mortality. Association with Age at Death and Compression of Mortality." *Journal of Clinical Epidemiology* Jul. 1992, 45(7): 733–42.

29. Demisch, L., Demisch, K., and Nickelsen, T. "Influence of Dexamethasone on Nocturnal Melatonin Production in Healthy Adult Subjects." *Journal of Pineal Research* 1988; 5: 317–22.

30. Touitou, Y., Fevre-Montagne, M., and Nakache, J.P. "Age and Sex-Associated Modification of Plasma Melatonin Concentrations in Man. Relationship to Pathology, Malignant or Not, and Autopsy Findings." *Acta Endocrinologica* 1985; 108: 135–44. Waldenlind, E., Wetterberg, L., and Filippi, U. "Lowered Circan-

nual Urinary Melatonin Concentrations in Episodic Cluster Headache." *Cephalalgia* 1994; 14: 199–204.

31. Waldenlind, E., Wetterberg, L., and Filippi, U. "Lowered Circannual Urinary Melatonin Concentrations in Episodic Cluster Headache." *Cephalalgia* 1994; 14: 199–204.

32. Doll, R., et al. "Mortality in Relation to Smoking: 40 Years' Observations on Male British Doctors." *British Medical Journal* 1994 Oct. 8; 309(6959): 901–11.

33. Ekman, A.C., Leppaluoto, J., and Vakkuri, O. "Ethanol Inhibits Melatonin Secretion in Healthy Volunteers in a Dose-Dependent Randomized Double Blind Cross-Over Study." *Journal of Clinical Endocrinology and Metabolism* 1993; 77: 780–83. The authors suggest that alcohol may disrupt melatonin production by lowering the body's level of tryptophan, the amino acid precursor of melatonin.

34. Rouhani, S., et al. "EEG Effects of a Single Low Dose of Ethanol on Afternoon Sleep in the Nonalcohol-Dependent Adult." *Alcohol* 1989 Jan.-Feb.; 6(1): 87–90.

35. Badia, P., Murphy, P.J., and Wright, K.P., Jr. "Alcohol Ingestion and Nighttime Melatonin Levels." *Sleep Research* 1994; 23: 477.

CHAPTER 16: CREATING A MELATONIN-FRIENDLY LIFESTYLE

1. Melatonin was identified in algae in 1991. In 1993 three botanists from the University of California at Davis, David Van Tassel, Juan Li, and Sharman O'Neill, identified melatonin in a higher plant, the Japanese morning glory. They are currently exploring the role that melatonin might play in triggering the flowering of photoperiodic plants.

2. Hattori, A., Migitakia, H., Reiter, R.J. "Identification of Melatonin in Plants and its Effects on Plasma Mel-

atonin Levels and Binding to Melatonin Receptors in Vertebrates." *Biochemistry and Molecular Biology International* 1995; 35: 627–34.

3. Hajak, G., Huether, G., Poeggeler, B., and Ruther, E. "The Influence of Intravenous L-Tryptophan on Plasma Melatonin and Sleep in Men." *Pharmacopsychiatry* 1991; 24: 17–20.

4. The contamination coincided with the introduction of a new bacterial strain used in the production of tryptophan. The impurity is believed to have been a product of the fermentation process.

5. Medsger, T.A., Jr. "Tryptophan-Induced Eosinophilia-Myalgia Syndrome." *New England Journal of Medicine* 1990; 322: 926–27.

6. Dakshinamurti, K., Paulose, C.S., and Sharma, S.K. "Neurobiology of Pyridoxine." *Annals of the New York Academy of Sciences* 1990; 585: 128–44.

7. Van den Berg, H., Bode, W., and Lowik, M.R. "Effect of Aging on Vitamin B-6 Status and Metabolism." *Annals of the New York Academy of Sciences* 1990; 5: 96–105.

8. Morton, D.J., Reiter, R.J. "Involvement of Calcium in Pineal Gland Function." *Society for Experimental Biology and Medicine*, 1991.

9. Vitamin B-6 (pyridoxine) can be toxic in high doses. Reports show that doses as low as 500 milligrams per day or even 200 milligrams can prove neurotoxic in some people. It is generally agreed that doses of 100 milligrams and less are safe for most adults.

10. Massion, A.O., Teas, J., and Kabat-Zinn, J. "Meditation, Melatonin and Breast/Prostate Cancer: Hypothesis and Preliminary Data." *Medical Hypotheses* 1995; 44: 39–46.

11. Lissoni, P., Resentini, M., and Fraschini, F. "Effects of Tetrahydrocannabinol on Melatonin Secretion in Man." *Hormone and Metabolic Research* 1986; 18: 77–78. At baseline, the mean value of their melatonin levels was 21.3 pg/ml. Two hours later, it was 904 pg/ml.

12. Grinspoon, L., and Bakalar, J.B. "Marihuana as Medicine." *Journal of the American Medical Association* 1995; 273(23): 1875–76.

CHAPTER 17: TAKING MELATONIN SUPPLEMENTS

1. Robert Sack, personal communication.
2. Nordlund, J.J., and Lerner, A.B. "The Effects of Oral Melatonin on Skin Color and on the Release of Pituitary Hormones." *Journal of Clinical Endocrinology and Metabolism* 1976; 45(4): 768–74.
3. Wright, J., Aldhous, M., and Arendt, J. "The Effect of Exogenous Melatonin on Endocrine Function in Man." *Clinical Endocrinology* 1986; 24: 375–82.
4. Kane, M.A., Johnson, A., and Robinson, W.A. "Serum Melatonin Levels in Melanoma Patients After Repeated Oral Administration." *Melanoma Research* 1994; 4: 59–65.
5. Terzolo, M., Piovesan, A., and Angeli, A. "Effects of Long-Term, Low-Dose, Time-Specified Melatonin Administration on Endocrine and Cardiovascular Variables in Adult Men." *Journal of Pineal Research* 1990; 9: 113–24.
6. Lissoni, P., Barni, S., Tancini, G., and Fraschini, F. "Clinical Study of Melatonin in Untreatable Advanced Cancer Patients." *Tumori* 1987; 73: 475–80.
7. Sakson, S. "New Tylenol Ads Stress Safety of Product but Not the Risks." Associated Press. *Oregonian*, Jan. 5, 1995, p. B-2.
8. Lewis, A.E. *KAL Center for Nutrition Research Bulletin*, July 23, 1995.
9. Maestroni, G.J., and Conti, A. "Anti-stress Role of the Melatonin-immuno-opioid Network: Evidence for a Physiological Mechanism Involving T-Cell-derived, Immunoreactive B-Endorphin and Metenkephalin Binding the Thymic Opioid Receptors." *International Journal of Neuroscience* 1991; 61: 289–98.

10. Voordouw, B., Euser, R., Verdonk, R., and Cohen, M. "Melatonin and Melatonin-Progestin Combinations Alter Pituitary-Ovarian Function in Women and Can Inhibit Ovulation." *Journal of Clinical Endocrinology and Metabolism* 1992; 74(1): 108–17.

11. Infants do not produce significant quantities of melatonin until the age of three or four months. There must be a reason for this phenomenon. I have suggested that melatonin may prevent the programmed death of brain neurons that occurs in the first few months of life, a part of the necessary reorganization of an infant's brain. Infants do get melatonin through the mother's breast milk, but if a nursing mother were to take exogenous melatonin, it would give her abnormally high levels of melatonin. What effects this would have on the child's development is unknown.

12. Carman, J.S., Post, R.M., and Goodwin, F.K. "Negative Effects of Melatonin on Depression." *American Journal of Psychiatry* 1976; 133(10): 1181–86.

13. A study just released, however, suggests that melatonin may be *helpful* for people with inflammatory diseases such as asthma and allergies. Melatonin down-regulates the gene that produces the enzyme 5-lipoxygenase. This enzyme catalzyes the production of a class of substances known as leukotrines, and leukotrines cause inflammatory reactions. Nonetheless, people with inflammatory diseases should wait for researchers to resolve these issues before taking melatonin. Steinhilber, D., Brungs, M., and Carlberg, C. "The Nuclear Receptor for Melatonin Represses 5-Lipoxygenase Gene Expression in Human B-Lymphocytes." *Journal of Biological Chemistry* 1995; 270(13): 7037–40.

14. Hansson, I., Holmdahl, R., Mattsson, R. "The Pineal Hormone Melatonin Exaggerates Development of Collagen-Induced Arthritis in Mice." *Journal of Neuroimmunology* 1992; 39: 23–30.

15. Georges Maestroni, personal communication.

16. Jan, J.E., Espezel, H., and Appleton, R.E. "The Treat-

ment of Sleep Disorders with Melatonin." *Developmental Medicine and Child Neurology* 1994; 36: 97–107.

17. To my knowledge, this type of atypical reaction has not been seen in clinical studies involving melatonin but only among members of the public who have taken commercially available melatonin in unsupervised situations. Thus the reaction may have to do with their underlying mental condition or a *negative* placebo effect.

18. Interestingly, for many years pineal researchers such as myself were given our melatonin free of charge, courtesy of the Nestlé company in Switzerland. Chemists at Nestlé had discovered that one of the by-products of their patented process for making decaffeinated coffee happened to be pure melatonin. Now that there is such a high demand for melatonin, we no longer get our melatonin gratis.

19. Before being excreted, the 6-hydroxymelatonin is conjugated to become either 6-hydroxymelatonin sulfate or 6-hydroxymelatonin-glucaronate, the actual substances that appear in the liver.

20. Aldhous, M., Franey, C., Arendt, J. "Plasma Concentrations of Melatonin in Man Following Oral Absorption of Different Preparations." *British Journal of Clinical Pharmacology* 1985; 19: 517–21.

21. Sandyk, R., Anninos, P.A., and Tsagas, N. "Age-Related Disruption of Circadian Rhythms: Possible Relationship to Memory Impairment and Implications for Therapy with Magnetic Fields." *International Journal of Neuroscience* 1991; 59: 259–62.

CHAPTER 18: WHEN GOD HOLDS THE PATENT

1. Loeb, S., ed. *Professional Guide to Diseases*. 4th ed. (Springhouse, PA: Springhouse Corp., 1992), p. 396.
2. Kulmann, G., Neri, F., and Lissoni, P. "Lack of Light/

Dark Rhythm of the Pineal Hormone Melatonin (MLT) in Autistic Children." Presented at the First International Congress of Clinical Neuroimmodulation. Monza, Italy, 1995.

3. Porter, R.J. *Epilepsy*. 1982. NIH publication 82–2369.

4. For a good review on the topic, see Champney, T.H., and Peterson, C., "Circadian, Seasonal, Pineal, and Melatonin Influences on Epilepsy." *Melatonin: Biosynthesis, Physiological Effects, and Clinical Applications* (Baton Rouge: CRC Press, 1993).

5. Fariello, R.G., Bubenik, A., Grota, L.J. "Epileptogenic Action of Intraventricularly Injected Antimelatonin Antibody." *Neurology* 1977; 27: 567–70. This study is regarded as more conclusive because the effect could not be attributed to the trauma of surgery. Also, the antibodies cause a greater reduction in melatonin than a pinealectomy, because some melatonin is produced in other parts of the body.

6. According to Anton-Tay's report, "Melatonin administration was followed by a progressive decrease in the amplitude of the electrical activity of the temporal lobe with a general tendency to the synchronization of the amygdala and the cortex. . . . Paroxistic EEG activity was markedly depressed during the first four hours following administration of the hormone."

7. Anton-Tay, F., Diaz, J.L., and Fernandez-Guardiola, A. "On the Effect of Melatonin Upon Human Brain. Its Possible Therapeutic Implications." *Life Sciences* 1971; 10(1): 841–50.

8. This case history is now being written up for publication by Acuña Castroviejo.

9. Ramaekers, V.T., Calomme, M., and Makropoulos, W. "Selenium Deficiency Triggering Intractable Seizures." *Neuropediatrics* 1994; 25: 217–23

10. Larry Sparks, personal communication. In 1988 he published his findings about a much smaller number of glands from SIDS infants. See Sparks, D.L., Hunsaker, J.C. "The Pineal Gland in Sudden Infant

Death Syndrome: Preliminary Observations." *Journal of Pineal Research* 1988; 5: 111–18.

11. Larry Sparks, personal communication. This data is soon to be published. Sparks reports that of 111 pineal glands of SIDS infants, only five were normal sized (P < 0.0001). Those five could be accounted for by misdiagnosis of the cause of death.

12. Wurtman, R.J., Lynch, H.J., and Sturner, W.Q. "Melatonin in Humans: Possible Involvement in SIDS, and Use in Contraceptives." *Advances in Pineal Research* 1991; 5: 319–26.

13. Sparks, L.D., and Hunsaker, J.C. "Increased ALZ-50—Reactive Neurons in the Brains of SIDS Infants: An Indicator of Greater Neuronal Death?" *Journal of Child Neurology* 1991; 6: 123–27. Sparks has found a significant increase in degenerating neurons in the hippocampus and medulla in SIDS infants compared with children who died from other causes (P < 0.0001).

14. O'Brien, I.A.D., Lewin, I.G., Arendt, J., and Corrall, R.J.M. "Abnormal Circadian Rhythm of Melatonin in Diabetic Autonomic Neuropathy." *Clinical Endocrinology* 1986; 24: 359–64. None of the three subjects with diabetic retinopathy, the authors note, had a melatonin rhythm. Is the altered melatonin rhythm in diabetics cause or effect? In terms of the patients with autonomic neuropathy, the authors suggest it could be the result of sympathetic denervation.

15. Sridhar, G.R. and Madhu, K. "Prevalence of Sleep Disturbances in Diabetes Mellitus." *Diabetes Research and Clinical Practice* 1994 Apr.; 23(3): 183–86.

16. Wolff, S.P. "Diabetes Mellitus and Free Radicals." *British Medical Bulletin* 1993; 49(3): 642–52.

17. Pierrefiche, G., Topall, G., Courboin, G., Henriet, I., and Laborit, H. "Antioxidant Activity of Melatonin in Mice." *Research Communications in Chemical Pathology and Pharmacology* 1993; 80(2): 211–23.

18. Champney, T.H., Brainard, G.C., and Reiter, R.J.

"Experimentally-Induced Diabetes Reduced Nocturnal Pineal Melatonin Content in the Syrian Hamster." *Comparative Biochemistry and Physiology* 1983; 76A(1): 199–201.

19. Rodriguez, V., Mellado, C., and Blazquez, E. "Effect of Pinealectomy on Liver Insulin and Glucagon Receptor Concentrations in the Rat." *Journal of Pineal Research* 1989; 6: 77–88.

20. Guardiola-Lemaitre, B. "Melatonin Agonist/Antagonist: From the Receptor to Therapeutic Applications." In *Advances in Pineal Research*, vol. 8, ed. M. Møller and P. Pévet (London: John Libbey and Co., 1994), pp. 333–48.

21. Eric Parker, personal communication.

22. Tan, D.-X., Chen, L.-D., and Reiter, R.J. "Melatonin: A Potent, Endogenous Hydroxyl Radical Scavenger." *Endocrine Journal* 1993; 1: 57–60.

RESOURCES

I've made a number of recommendations throughout the book for a melatonin-friendly lifestyle. The following is a list of products and professional services that might also help you achieve this goal.

MELATONIN SUPPLIERS

Dozens of companies are now offering melatonin for sale. The following is a list of suppliers that have told us they conduct independent assays of the purity of their melatonin. (This list is not meant to imply that a number of other companies lack similar quality-control standards.)

Life Extension Foundation
P.O. Box 229120
Hollywood, FL 33022-9120
(800) 841-5433
(305) 966-4886 (other countries)
Method of Payment: Visa/MasterCard, Discover, C.O.D. (for an additional shipping charge). *Available doses: 0.5 mg., 1 mg., 3 mg., 10 mg. (60 capsules per bottle), plus a 3 mg. timed-release formulation.*

Wholesale Nutrition
P.O. Box 3345
Saratoga, CA 95070
(800) 325-2664 (U.S. and Canada)

(408) 867-6368 (other countries)
Available doses: 3 mg. tablets (sublingual), 400 per bottle.

Nutricology
400 Preda Street
San Leandro, CA 94577
(800) 545-9960 (U.S. and Canada)
(510) 639-4572 (other countries)
(510) 635-6730 (fax)
  Method of Payment: Check, money order, Visa/Master-Card, letter of credit, credit account with prior approval. *Available doses: 20 mg., 3 mg., 1.3 mg., 300 micrograms (0.3 mg.) and a 1.2 mg. time-release formulation.* Variable quantities available, call for more information.

Cardiovascular Research
1061-B Shary Circle
Concord, CA 94518
(800) 888-4585 U.S. and Canada
(510) 827-2636 (other countries)
  Method of payment: Check, Visa/MasterCard, C.O.D. *Available doses 0.5 mg., 3 mg., 10 mg., and a 1.8 mg. sustained release formulation.*

PHYSICIANS AND CLINICS

For help with sleep problems, I suggest that you call a sleep disorders clinic in your area. An increasing number of sleep disorder specialists are now prescribing melatonin to their patients. You can write to the following address for more information:

National Sleep Foundation
1367 Connecticut Avenue, N.W.
Washington, D.C. 20036
  At this time only a limited number of physicians, psychologists, and other health professionals have adequate

knowledge of melatonin or clinical experience in recommending and monitoring its use for the other health problems and diseases I've talked about in this book. The following health professionals have used melatonin in clinical practice.

Sarafina Corsella, M.D.
200 W. 57th St.
New York, NY 10019
Dr. Corsella is a psychiatrist in private practice in Huntington, Long Island, and in New York City. She has used melatonin to treat patients with PMS, endometriosis, and circadian-rhythm disorders.

Pain and Stress Therapy Center
5282 Medical Drive, Suite 160
San Antonio, TX 78229-6043
(210) 614-7246
The health professionals at the Pain and Stress Therapy Center work with patients seeking help with chronic pain, stress, depression, grief, anxiety, sleep difficulties, and PMS. They have recommended melatonin to hundreds of patients.

Whitaker Wellness Center
4321 Birch, Suite 100
Newport Beach, CA 92660
(714) 851-1550
More than twelve thousand patients have been treated at the Whitaker Wellness Center for treatment and prevention of arthritis, heart disease, high blood pressure, obesity, diabetes, chronic fatigue, and depression. Melatonin therapy may be part of a comprehensive overall program. For information about books by Dr. Julian Whitaker and the *Health & Healing* newsletter, call 1-800-777-5005.

LIGHT BOXES AND RELATED PRODUCTS

If you would like to increase your exposure to light during your waking hours, the following products will help.

MedEd Publications
P.O. Box 12415
Columbus, OH 43212
Write to this address for a consumer's guide to light therapy devices.

Apollo Light Systems
352 West 1060 Street
Orem, UT 84058
(801) 226-2370
Apollo Light Systems manufactures the Brite Lite III 10,000 lux box, Travel Lite 10,000 lux portable box, and a dawn simulator (a light that comes on gradually, mimicking the sunrise, to serve as a morning alarm clock).

Bio-Brite, Inc.
7315 Wisconsin Avenue, Suite 1300W
Bethesda, MD 20814-3202
(800) 621-LITE (U.S. and Canada)
(301) 961-8551 (other countries)
Bio-Brite provides a number of products to help relieve the symptoms of jet lag. Products include the Jet Lag Kit and the Jet Lag Calculator. They also have a dawn simulator (The SunRise Clock) and a Deluxe Light Visor, which is a light source that you wear on your head, essentially a portable light box. Bio-Brite makes a thirty-day rental available for the Jet Lag Kit.

Lighting Resources
1421 West Third Avenue
Columbus, OH 43212-2928
(800) 875-8489 or (614) 488-6841
Lighting Resources offers the Ultralight, Solar Plus, and

SunDial light boxes. They also manufacture The Light Hat, a device that fits on the brim of a baseball-style cap or visor.

Pi Square, Inc.
11036 First Avenue South
Seattle, WA 98168
(800) 786-3296 (800 SUN DAWN)
(206) 246-1101

Pi Square offers the SunUp and SunRizr dawn/dusk simulator as well as SunBox light boxes and track lighting systems. Light boxes include both desk and floor units and are rated at 10,000 lux.

EMF DETECTORS AND RELATED PRODUCTS

The following companies manufacture products designed to help you minimize your exposure to electromagnetic fields.

American Waterbed Wholesalers
10 Stage Door Road
Wappingers Falls, NY 12590
(800) 992-0373

This company manufactures a thermal waterbed liner that can take the place of the electrical heating unit. Not recommended for damp, cool climates. It can be used in conjunction with a heater. (Turn the heater on in the daytime, turn it off when you go to bed, and the liner will preserve the heat throughout the night.)

No Rad, Inc.
1160 East Sandhill Avenue
Carson, CA 90746
(310) 605-0808

No Rad manufactures electromagnetic field shield products for computer screens. When ordering, you will need the measurements of the entire monitor, including the diagonal measurement of the screen itself. They also manufacture an electric field meter, model 8100, that measures electric fields generated by video display terminals, AC power lines, and other electrical equipment.

Walker Scientific, Inc.
Rockdale Street
Worcester, MA 01606
(508) 852-3674

Walker Scientific manufactures various handheld instruments to measure low-level electromagnetic field radiation in the ELF and VLF frequency ranges. (For household use, we recommend the 60D model with a bandwidth of 40Hz to 400Hz.)

INDEX

ABOUT THE AUTHORS

RUSSEL J. REITER, PH.D., professor of neuroendocrinology at the University of Texas Health Science Center at San Antonio, received his Ph.D. in endocrinology from the Bowman Gray School of Medicine at Wake Forest University in 1964. In the subsequent thirty years he has received more than forty honors and awards, including two honorary doctorates in medicine and the coveted McIntyre Medal for Achievement in Medical Science.

Reiter is founder and editor-in-chief of *The Journal of Pineal Research*, and he has served on the advisory board of twenty-three other medical journals.

He is a member of many prestigious scientific organizations, including the New York National Academy of Science, the American Aging Association, the International Brain Research Organization, and the European Pineal Association.

Reiter has been first author or made substantial contributions to more than seven hundred research articles in peer-reviewed journals including *Science*, *Nature*, and *Lancet*. He has written six professional books and edited three others. He is also a dedicated teacher. He has worked with more than ninety postdoctoral students, many of them from outside the United States, and his outstanding teaching ability has earned him four separate citations.

JO ROBINSON is a medical writer from Portland, Oregon. She ferreted out the melatonin story while it was still hidden in obscure medical journals and spent a year interviewing scientists from around the world. The trail of evidence led her, ultimately, to Reiter's laboratory in Texas.

Robinson has collaborated on seven nonfiction books, including the best-selling *Getting the Love You Want* by Harville Hendrix. More than one million copies of her books have been sold.